AUTOPHAGY:

INCREASE SELF-CLEANSING METABOLIC PROCESS AND PROMOTE LONGEVITY. A SIMPLE DIET TO FAT BURN, LIVE HEALTHY AND LONGER WITH AUTOPHAGY.

DAN COOK

Table of Contents

Introduction

The cell itself will then recycle useful chemical components for other purposes. This process then allows for autophagy to adjust the stability of protein composition within a cell in our body. This helps to prevent the building up of toxic waste products, aids in sustaining cells during periods in which our body is starving, gets rid of invading pathogens, and maintains cellular organelle function.

Consider autophagy to be when your body creates a dumpster, also known as your autophagosome. What it does is collect cellular components and takes them to the local cellular "recycling center" which is scientifically known as the lysosome. This is where it gets broken down into small parts which are then repurposed into new pieces of machinery. New cells.

What is Autophagy?

A process that is very similar to it is called apoptosis, which is also known as "programmed cell death." After a set amount of time dividing, the cells are programmed to perish. This process may sound disturbing at first, but it is actually crucial in keeping a healthy body. For instance, consider it like having a vehicle. You buy it, you grow to adore it, and you create memories with it. It is a part of your life, and you take it places. However, as the years go by, your car naturally suffers wear and tear. After a while, as much as you love it, you have to let it go because it's eventually going to take a lot of money to keep it going. Moreover, even with the maintenance, your car breaks down continuously. You'll have to finally get another one because it's eventually leading to the junkyard. You don't want to keep it around by the time it becomes something that'll sit in your backyard, so you end up getting rid of it. You then got out and purchase a new one.

This analogy helps us to understand what's going on in our bodies. Our cells slowly become useless and old. It is ideal for them to be programmed to die when they no longer can do what they were built to do in the first place. This is what science calls "apoptosis." Cells are destined to die before they're even born, that is after they've exhausted their usefulness. Taking it back to our car analogy, after a certain time has past and our car is no longer able to work, and then we get a new one. The good news with this process though is that you don't have to worry about having to "purchase" anything. With autophagy, your body will do it on its own.

When our bodies are running well, and the cells are running smoothly, autophagy happens at a lower level, which helps us recycle these worn-down cellular mechanisms. We're in a good maintenance mode. Things can become complicated when they're stressed, however. In the cellular scenario, stress comes from when our bodies don't have enough nutrients or energy, from un-recycled and dysfunctional components, or when microbes invade them. Autophagy then gets "turned up" because it's going to work to help save us. Science calls this the "stress mode."

This process also happens in what science calls the sub-cellular level. Returning to the car analogy, you don't really have to get rid of the entire car, per se. At the time, all you need to do is replace a part, like putting in a new battery. Out with the old and in with the new! The killing off the entire cell is what makes apoptosis different from autophagy. For the process of autophagy, the sub-cellular organelles are killed off, and new ones are rebuilt to take over for the old ones. Organelles, old cell membranes, and other parts of a cell that are cast-off are able to be removed. This happens by transferring it to the lysosome which is an organelle that contains enzymes that help to degrade proteins.

One thing that makes autophagy so remarkable is the process is in which it occurs happens when there is what science calls cellular stress. That is if the cells lack specific nutrients, or they are deprived of energy or become damaged for some reason, the "stress response" is activated and autophagy happens at a higher speed. This causes cell function to improve when we, and thus our bodies, are under duress. We'll explore more of this phenomenon in chapters two and four.

Ultimately, the science revolving around autophagy tells us is that it helps to make our bodies work better. By clearing out all of the cellular "junk" within us, we are

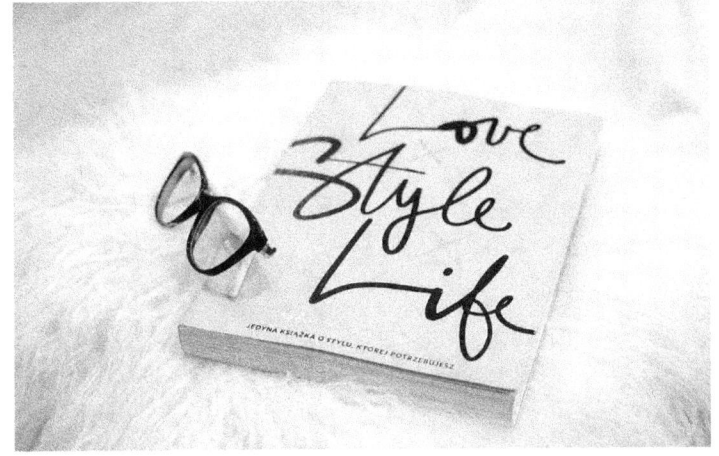

then clearing a way for cells to recreate themselves with new components. This biological upgrade can be seen as giving our car a new engine. It helps to keep us "running."

Chapter 1 Autophagy Benefits

Autophagy is one of the most critical processes for our health. In simple terms, the garbage collection cleans the body and cleanses the cells. Autophagy ensures that metabolic waste products and other weak cells are broken down and recycled. That's hugely important to our health.

Autophagy is able to delay physical and mental aging, prevent cancer, prevent the growth of tumors in early stages or prevent neurodegenerative diseases such as Alzheimer's.

But it goes much further: imagine that instead of defective parts of the same cell are VIRUSES, BACTERIA, FUNGI that are captured for their elimination.

Autophagy helps you fight the infection. Listen to your body and let it do its job.

I invite you to remember the last time you were very sick. I will also remind you that you knew that you were because even though you are "good tooth" HUNGER WAS REMOVED. I will also remind you that within 2-3 days you knew that you were recovering when the hunger came back. But you were more focused on listening to your mother, neighbors, friends, who urged you to eat to RECOVER FASTER when your body was telling you. LET ME FOCUS ON GETTING OUT THIS INFECTION and then you'll be fine.

Autophagy can help you reduce excess skin product of massive weight loss

Intermittent fasting and insulin resistance helps you lose weight, you see that the body is a perfect machine and, if you learn to listen and take care of it, not only will you lose weight, but that skin surplus will decrease.

Autophagy can improve your digestion

Inducing autophagy by fasting puts your digestive system at rest. It allows the gastrointestinal tract to relax, which helps decrease inflammation and improves intestinal motility. It also improves the absorption of nutrients and stimulates the growth of good bacteria in your intestine.

It also helps cardiovascular health

Autophagy can reduce heart rate and blood pressure. The strength of your cardiovascular system improves after inducing autophagy. Some studies have been able to prove this, but the exact mechanism is not yet clear.

Anti-aging

Fasting and exercise are sometimes the best means of anti-aging, not only because of increased secretion of growth hormone but also because of autophagy. Damaged or weak cells are broken down and replaced with new cells. This applies to cells of all kinds and slows down aging in some ways.

Immune system

Autophagy breaks down and destroys viruses, bacteria, and other pathogens in the cells. This strengthens the autophagy of our immune system and supports this in the defense against pathogens. This is sometimes a reason why we usually feel little to no hunger during illness. The body signals that it does not want food to get into autophagy. Thus, the immune system can work better, and the body heals faster. This is sometimes the reason why fasting is so effective against so many diseases. It strengthens the immune system in a natural way.

Brain Health

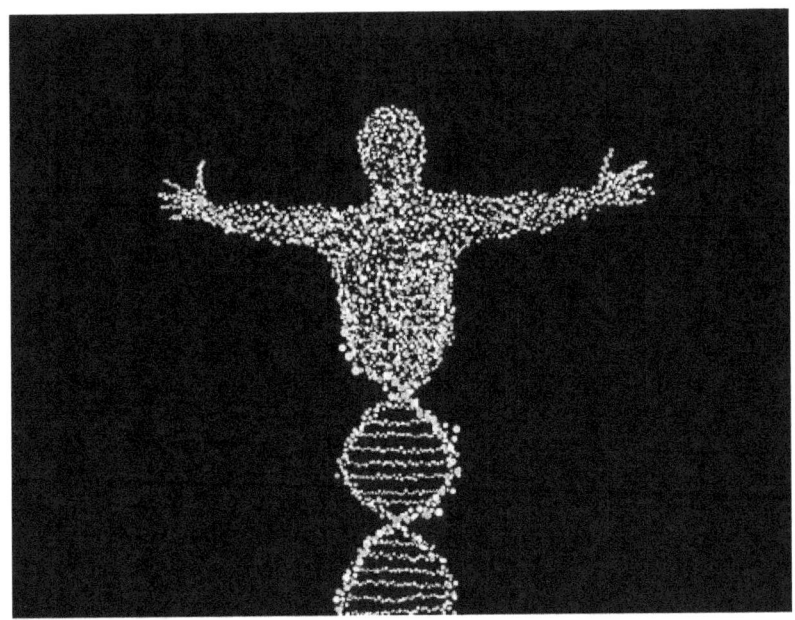

Another important point the researchers have been able to confirm is the effect against dementia, Parkinson's, and other brain disorders. Although the origins may be different, an accumulation of misfolded proteins is usually the cause. These accumulate in the course of life but can be effectively degraded and recycled by autophagy. Thus, autophagy protects both preventively and treated against numerous brain diseases.

Researchers were able to demonstrate this effect, inter alia, by the administration of spermidine. This ingredient comes in varying concentrations in different foods and has been proven to boost autophagy. This, in turn, had a positive effect on numerous symptoms and diseases.

Chapter 2 Myths vs. Truths

Before we get into more information about fasting and what it all entails, it is important to dispel some of the common myths and misconceptions that can come with the idea of fasting and autophagy. These misconceptions are going to make it hard to convince some people that going on a fast is actually a good idea. We have spent years hearing about how we need to eat every few hours and that skipping meals is such a bad thing for us – when, in reality, it can help to speed up our metabolisms and the process of autophagy.

Let's take a look at some of the most common myths that are out there about fasting and autophagy and come to understand why they are instead really good for our overall health.

Fasting Is Going to Put Your Body in Starvation Mode

One common misconception that many people will have when it comes to going on a fast is that fasting will put you into starvation mode. Starvation mode is the period in your body where the metabolism shuts down to conserve energy because you have gone a long time without food. If starvation mode occurs too much, it can mess with the metabolism and make weight loss almost impossible.

However, for the most part, unless you do something really off with your fast, you will see some amazing benefits when you go on a fast, without ever having to worry about going into starvation mode at the same time. Most research shows that it takes at least 72 hours before starvation mode becomes a big problem for most people. Since many people decide that they will stick with intermittent fasting, they will be on and off the fast before these issues even come up.

Even if you do go on a longer fast, as long as you aren't fasting all of the time, and you eat a healthy diet beforehand, you don't have to worry about starvation mode. Starvation mode is only going to be an issue when the individual decides to go on a fast for a very long time, or they go too extreme with their fasting rules. For example, if you go on a two-week fast every month and then cut your calories down to 800 for the rest of the month, you are probably not giving the body the nutrients it needs. If you go on a twenty-hour fast each day, and then only eat 500 calories after that, then there are issues as well.

The most important thing to remember about the starvation mode is that the body needs to feel that it is really short on nutrients and that it is likely not to get those nutrients soon. It goes into this mode as a way to deal with the lack of nutrients. If you keep your fasts reasonable, and make sure that you take in enough calories each day, or overall, with healthy and nutritious foods, then you can enjoy going on a fast and experiencing the autophagic process, without having to worry about starvation mode.

Fasting Is Going to Make You Overeat and Can Ruin the Effects of Autophagy

One common concern that comes up when we talk about fasting and autophagy is the idea that once you are done with the fast, you are going to overeat, and then all of the benefits will be canceled out. It is true that you are going to be incredibly hungry when you are done with fasting; however, this doesn't mean that you have to give in to those cravings and those urges along the way.

This is where some planning needs to come in. You may have the best resolution in the world to not overeat and to stay healthy and get all of the benefits from fasting, but then you go some time without eating, and you get hungry. When you're eating window finally opens again, you are going to be really hungry, and your body will crave everything sweet and unhealthy. Without some planning, it is possible that you will end up overeating.

This doesn't mean that you are counteracting all the benefits of the autophagy that occurred during that time. However, it is something that you need to work on a bit. Meal planning can definitely be the answer that you are looking for if you decide to go on a fast to help with weight loss as well.

When you come up with a meal plan, consider adding a few extra calories into the beginning meal, or the first

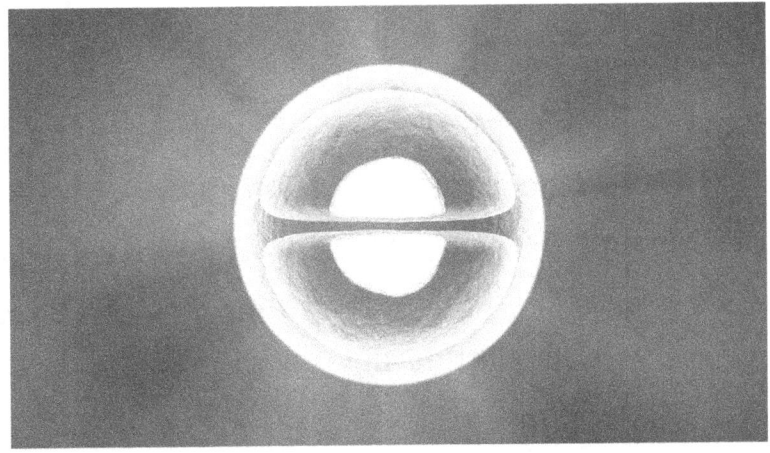

one that you have after you finish the fast. And perhaps consider having a healthier "treat" on there. In the beginning, you are going to have cravings, and they will be hard to deal with. And you are going to be hungry. Don't ignore this. Rather than trying to split up the calories completely even when you have three meals after the fast, give the first meal some extra calories, and cut the others down a little bit. This helps you to eat a little extra and satisfy those cravings, while also ensuring that you aren't going to feel deprived.

Fasting Is Bad for Your Health

We have had some long-held beliefs that fasting is a horrible thing for our bodies. We assume that it is going to put our bodies into starvation mode, that we are going to feel miserable, and that we will have such a slow metabolism from missing even one meal that we can kiss losing weight goodbye forever.

But does any of this really make sense? Does it make sense that we would enter starvation mode just from missing a meal or two? Our ancestors didn't have a ton of food just sitting around, and they may have had to go several days without getting any good at all. Does this mean that they went into starvation mode and their metabolisms were ruined all the time?

Have you ever been sick and had to go a few days without eating? Whether you were just suffering from the flu and didn't have anything to eat for a few days, or you were throwing up and couldn't keep anything down, we have all

gone without eating during that time as well. Did that mean we entered into starvation mode and our metabolisms were ruined forever?

Of course not. Our bodies are designed to take a little bit of stress and missing a meal here or there is not a big deal. Studies and research have shown that you can go up to 72 hours on a fast before the big side effects of starvation mode start to become an issue. And as long as you make sure that your diet is full of healthy and nutritious foods when you are no longer fasting, it is easy to add in the daily, or a few times a week, fasts that are common with intermittent fasting.

If you can add one of the protocols of fasting into your routine, you are going to get a whole host of benefits out of the process. You will get to enjoy a healthier heart, weight loss, mental clarity, better blood pressure, fewer issues with insulin resistance and diabetes, and so much more – all it takes it putting the body on a short fast on occasion and allowing the process of autophagy to take control.

Fasting and Autophagy Will Burn Off Muscles

Studies that take a look at alternate daily fasting show that the concern over losing muscle on a fast is misplaced. Alternate daily fasting over a period that was 70 days long did see a decrease in body weight of an average of six percent in participants. However, the fat mass of those same individuals did increase by eleven-point four percent. But the lean mass, which includes muscle and bone, didn't see any changes at all.

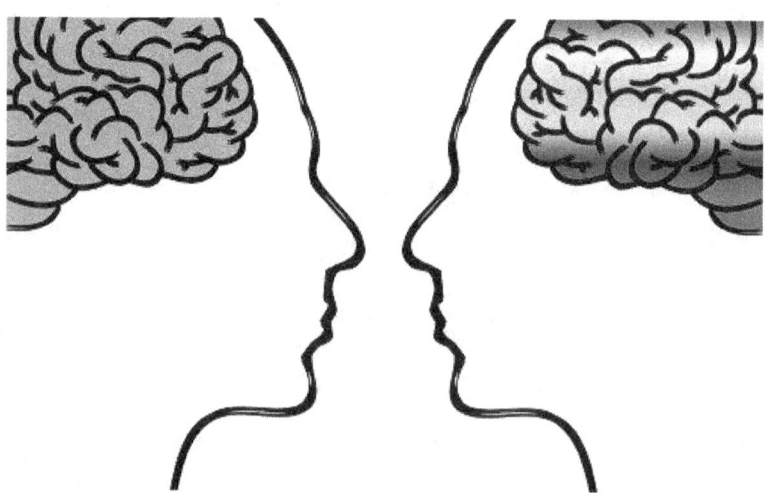

In addition, there were big improvements that were seen in the LDL (low-density lipoprotein) and triglyceride

levels. The growth hormone increased, which was important in helping the participants maintain their muscle mass. To take this even further, some studies show that eating just one meal each day resulted in a significant amount of fat loss, even if that meal included the same number of calories as eating three or more times during the day. The most important thing here, though, is that there was no evidence of muscle loss at all.

Let's take this even further. More recently, a randomized trial of fasting versus caloric restriction found that there really wasn't any evidence that muscle was burned up during the fasting process. During this same trial, the fasting group was told to follow the 36-hour fasting protocol every other day, also known as alternate day fasting. This shows great promise for those who want to get started on fasting for all of the health benefits, but who were scared about the loss in the muscle that may result.

According to some experts who seem not to look at the studies above, fasting will burn off 1/3 of a pound of muscle each day that you are on it. What this results in is about 1 pound of muscle a week if you go on an alternate day fast. This also means that you would see a reduction of 32 pounds of muscle in a group that does fasting for 32 weeks.

However, the actual amount that the fasting group lost over 32 weeks was about 2.6 pounds or 1.2 kg. Yes, this was a little bit of muscle weight loss, but when it was compared to the participants who just went on a calorie restriction, it was less. Those participants who simply restricted their calories ended up losing 16 kg during that same period.

It makes sense that a bit of lean mass is going to be lost when you lose weight. You are losing some of the extra skin and connective tissue at the same time, but the lean mass percentage actually does increase by about 22 percent when you are on a fast.

As you can see, fasting does not burn off a ton of muscle mass, and it won't make you a weak person who is going to suffer from metabolism issues for the rest of your life because you no longer have any muscle mass to deal with. And if you are worried about the slight amount of muscle mass that is lost (which is still less than what you would see with just going on a calorie restriction), then consider adding in some strength training or weight training to your routine to help.

You Can't Exercise When You Are on a Fast

Another misconception is the idea that you are not allowed to work out when fasting. While it is true that you may have to go through and make some adjustments to the way that your workout compared to your normal routine, this doesn't mean that you aren't allowed to work out at all.

When you go on a fast, you are working to deplete the stores of glycogen that are in the body so that you start relying more on the stored fat. During this process, the body may feel a little bit tired and worn down. It is so used to getting the glycogen on a regular basis, and that is a much easier source of fuel for it to rely on than the stored fat. The body will feel weak and worn down for a few days, and sometimes even later on as it adjusts to the fasting regimen.

Because of this, you may need to make some changes to the way that you exercise. Doing the workout right at the beginning of the fast can help because it ensures that you still have some glucose floating around the body to give you energy. Switching to something like HIIT training or weightlifting can be a nice way to ensure that you are still getting a good workout, that you are working on building and maintaining those strong muscles, and that you see even better results from both the fast and autophagy.

Autophagy Means We Have to Overstress Our Bodies

When it comes to autophagy, it is true that the body needs to undergo some stress to make the process happen. This is critical to assuring that the body will start to break down the old parts and build up new ones. If there is no breaking down, then how will there be room for the new cells and parts that you need?

This doesn't mean that we have to overstress our bodies and go crazy. Doing workouts that last six or seven hours each day and are incredibly intense or fasting for a month straight may seem like they will help out more, but you will find that there are actually more effective, and easier, methods for starting the body on this process.

Simple exercise, such as an intense 30-minute workout or HIIT training, can be enough to help when you are looking to enter into autophagy. Going on a fast that is a few days long, or even just a one-day fast, can be enough to get the body started with autophagy. And these are much easier to start and maintain compared to the more intense options above. Autophagy needs a bit of stress to get started, but that doesn't mean that you have to go crazy in order to see the results.

Autophagy can be a great process for your whole body. It ensures that the body can function properly because it gets all of those old cells and proteins and other parts and removes them so that new ones can start. It is a simple concept to work with, but you will find that it really does make a difference throughout your whole body.

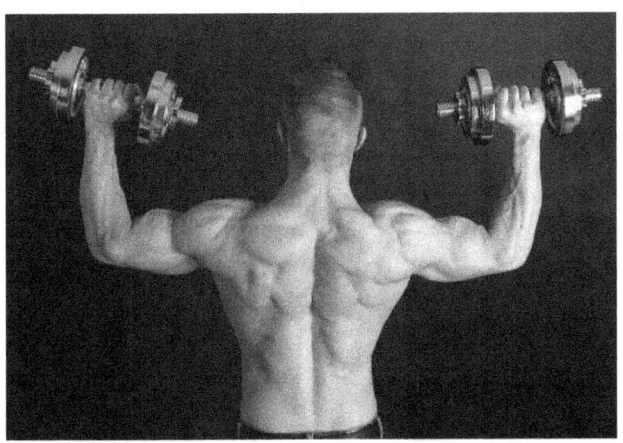

Chapter 3 Autophagy Performance

The answer to autophagy is in the question of how you want to look at your own health and healing. Too many people are trying to perform at the same level using the same tricks of the trade, flopping back and forth between all of the culturally popular diet crazes, and falling off the wagon on account of highs, lows, and cravings. If you understand how autophagy works, then you also understand that to look at it from the point of view of universal success isn't going to work.

Yes, all of our cells have the same function of cell renewal and autophagy, but no one has the same genetic make-up, DNA, and body type. We can't all fit into the same box, which is why you need to resist the tendency to adopt the program that everyone else is using. We don't have the same reasons for going on diets, exercising, and looking for a cure to health problems. From an outside point of view, it can look the same: weight loss, bigger muscles, long life. However, tapping into the reality of autophagy means truly looking at and listening to your body wisdom.

You are going to heal under the right circumstances for you, but what are those conditions? You can't take the exact same routine from your neighbor and expect the same results; it just doesn't work that way. In order to see a true turn around in your health, you have to tinker with the plan for healing that is unique to you.

Following the instructions of any diet, weight loss, and exercise program can feel like a lot of work. When you fall, of course, there can be a lot of doubt and discouragement that leads to continuing old patterns of eating and digesting. What you get out of autophagy is so much more than the common weight loss program, because it isn't just about weight loss and muscle building; it's about deep cellular healing for long-lasting life.

Because our culture stresses all of the weight loss routines and breaking bad habits, we find ourselves pigeon-holed into dieting in short-lived spurts for short term effect, rather than altering the concept of our internal workings and changing our bodies from deep within on the microscopic level. It isn't just how you look on the outside; it's how you feel deep within and how your cells perform and function.

Creating autophagy for health benefits isn't hard. It's not a gimmick or a fad; it's your body intelligence working for you behind the scenes, and all you have to do is create the right conditions for that to occur. You may find some general theories and practices in this book that can help you get started with your renewal program; however, so much of the experience is going to be your own awareness of how your body works and how it doesn't. Your heredity can play a big part in your body structure and body top, meaning that not everyone will look the same when they lose 30 pounds.

Our anatomy is based on the same principles of structure and function that clean and heals us constantly, without obvious notice, but if we are not doing the work to create those circumstances, how can we put that gift to the test? Bringing autophagy to the foreground in your food intake, fasting and exercise cycles can change your whole health and reality.

This chapter will go into greater detail what you can do specifically to enact autophagy through guidelines and steps to understanding each diet, fast and muscle performance so you can fine-tune the healing experience that is right for you.

Weight loss occurs for everyone differently. We all have our genetic background, healthy or unhealthy eating habits and a long list of favorite snacks and treats that we go, for when we need an exciting pick-me-up. On the day to day level, we pick and graze between meals and have an endless number of options to choose from at the grocery store and restaurants. Many of us enjoy a large number of carbohydrates, delicious sugary food and drink, and a hearty helping of premade convenience foods regularly.

All of these factors, from the dietary standpoint, are what lead to the internal cell deficiency that autophagy works to heal. Because we all have our unique internal make-up, it is important to listen to our bodies when beginning to shift into ketosis diets, or keto-diets, as they are often called.

There are side effects of starting ketosis that can cause flu-like feelings that will discourage the continuation of the diet. Often times, these symptoms are the result of changing too much, too soon and can be prevented by gently easing into a change in diet, rather than going from zero to 100 mph.

What you can do is slowly start eliminating certain foods one day at a time to control your body's release of toxins. This tactic is known as partial elimination of these problematic foods. Ranging from days to weeks, careful elimination of these foods will lead to a healthier experience when adopting a new eating plan. Slow adaptation to this new diet will have fewer unpleasant side effects when approached in this way.

Most ketosis diets are relatively similar, but there are a few to consider when looking to create autophagy. They are:

- *Standard Keto Diet* (*75-20-5*)—This diet involves a ratio of fat to protein to carbohydrates, like the other keto diets will; however, the ratio in this diet usually creates the most noticeable change in the body resulting from fat loss and has a more profound impact overall on activating autophagy. The ratio is 75 percent fat, 20 percent protein, and 5 percent carbohydrates (75-20-5 daily intake). Keep in mind that based on your BMI, or body mass index, the measurements for these amounts will be different from person to person. If you weigh 160 lbs., versus someone who weighs 260, you will need to account for some change in measurement regarding the quantity of food, keeping the overall percentage of daily intake the same.

- *High Protein Keto Diet* (60-35-5)—This diet is similar to the standard keto diet, the only difference being the ratio shift. Rather than consuming 75 percent fat, it drops down to 60 percent, allowing for a higher percentage of protein daily. The reason someone might choose this ratio is if they are working to promote more muscle building rather than fat loss. For some people, starting with the standard diet helps them shave off the fat pounds, and once they have reached that goal they continue the keto diet, shifting to a high protein diet to help build muscle, especially if there isn't a large number of fat stores to burn.

- *Cyclical Keto Diet* (5:2)—Like with a 5:2 fasting ratio, this keto diet applies a method for exchanging fats for carbs on a 5 to 2 basis. For the first five days, you will eat a standard ketosis diet. For the following two days, you switch the ratio so that instead of high fat you are eating high carb (70-75% carb, 20-25% protein, 5-10% fat). This diet is often utilized for high-performance athletes who need a major carb load for weightlifting or workouts. It helps to create a balanced fat loss while building muscle mass.

- Targeted Keto Diet (carbs before exercise)— *This diet is like a hybrid diet of the standard and the cyclical keto diets. You maintain a typical standard keto diet and digest your daily carb allotment half an hour before your workout, allowing for muscle building and stamina in the workout without taking time off of ketosis.*

For the best results for autophagy performance, the standard and high protein diets are the best choices for creating ketosis and initiating an autophagic response. The other two diets may be more beneficial on a long-term track and should be considered, especially if you are a bodybuilder or athlete that requires more carb intake for building muscle and using energy.

Looking at the standard ketosis diet, you find the ratio of 75 percent fat, 20 percent protein, and 5 percent carbohydrate. Since the diet has almost no carbs, it is essential to start with partial elimination in a week to help avoid those uncomfortable flu-like symptoms. Once you fully eliminate carbs, you can pursue the standard ketosis diet regularly to increase your autophagic performance and overall body health. Some of the foods you will need to avoid eating on the standard ketosis diet are:

- *Sugar*—sweets, candy, juice, soda, energy drinks, sugar additives
- *Grains*—bread, pasta, cereal, rice, etc.
- *Starchy Vegetables*—root vegetables like beets, carrots, parsnips, potatoes, yams
- *Legumes*—Lentils, beans, chickpeas, peas
- *Fruit*—all fruit except small amounts of berries
- *Unhealthy Fats*—canola oil, vegetable oil, margarine, Crisco
- *Some condiments*—condiments that contain any of the above ingredients and especially store-bought mayonnaise
- *Low-Fat food products*—any packaged food that is marketed as being low fat
- Alcohol

Foods that you can enjoy on the standard ketosis diet:

- *Meat*—grass-fed beef, pork, poultry
- *Fish*—salmon, cod, tilapia
- *Eggs*
- *Dairy*—butter, cream, some cheeses
- *Nuts* and *seeds*
- *Healthy oils*—olive oil, coconut oil, avocado oil
- *Avocados*
- *Low-Carb Vegetables*—leafy greens, lettuce, peppers, tomatoes, onion, cucumbers, asparagus
- Herbs and Spices—*salt and pepper and a variety of herbs*

The standard diet may seem like it contains very limited ingredients; however, these simple foods can be arranged in countless delicious ways, and there are several delicious recipes specifically for ketosis diets that support this style of eating to support you along the way.

The ratio of foods in the standard diet is that you would have the highest amount of fat, allowing your body to run on fat stores instead of carbohydrates. While burning fat and experiencing ketosis, you ensure a healthy amount of protein so that you don't start eating your muscular protein in the process.

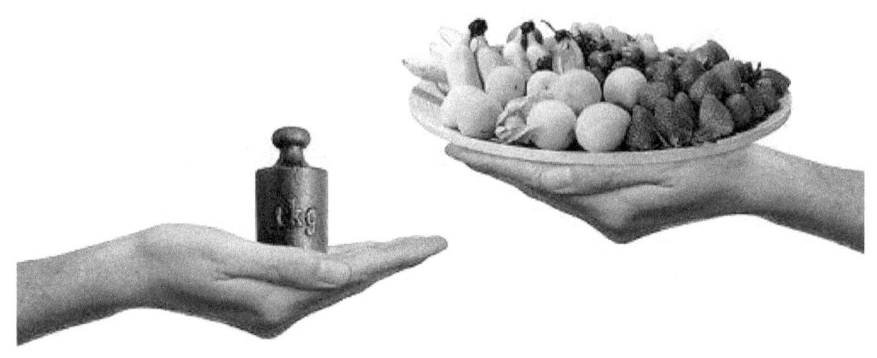

The alternative to that is the high protein version in which you slightly decrease the amount of fat, and increase the amount of protein, leaving the carbohydrate intake the same. The fat ratio goes down to 60 percent with the protein up to 35 percent, leaving the last 5 out of 100 for the carbs. You may elect this method if losing muscle mass is of greater concern, or if you are working on building muscle through ketosis.

The important aspect of why ketosis diets work is that with the high fat-high protein approach, your body will always feel full and satisfied. You will not crave treats, carbs or sugars, especially if you start with partial elimination of these foods before fully eliminating them from a standard ketosis diet. Many of the diets marketed today don't work because of this issue: cravings.

Cravings break the diet and cause a return to the same patterns of insulin resistance and high blood sugar.

It is important that if you choose a ketosis diet for encouraging autophagy performance, you must not eat high fat-high carbohydrate-high sugar. This is the recipe for obesity, diabetes, and countless other diseases of the body.

The necessary program for you is something you will need to tweak along the way, depending on your level of physical activity and your overall goal for health. The ketosis diets are one part of a system that aids in the control of autophagy performance. As you start to incorporate this kind of diet, you can begin adding in intermittent fasts that will continue to offer your body greater opportunity to heal on a cellular level.

Steps to Water Fasting

Controlling autophagy can be easy and pleasant with the right approach. After reading about ketosis diets to get you on the right track for autophagy regarding food intake, you can now begin to introduce a greater autophagic response by starting a fast. Plan on giving yourself a couple of months on a new diet before diving into a fast. Allowing time for your body to adjust to anything is healthy. There are some serious key components to consider as well as some precautions and contraindications, before getting started with the steps to water fasting.

When you are considering your water fast, it is important to plan ahead. You don't want to wake up one morning and casually decide that today is the day you aren't going to eat and only drink water (unless you are sick and know that it is necessary). A healthy fast requires preparation and planning and the slow tapering off of food intake.

If you have never fasted, or water fasted before, start with only one day of water only, or try the 16:8 fast. If you are doing a 16:8 fast, you won't need to worry as much about the following steps.

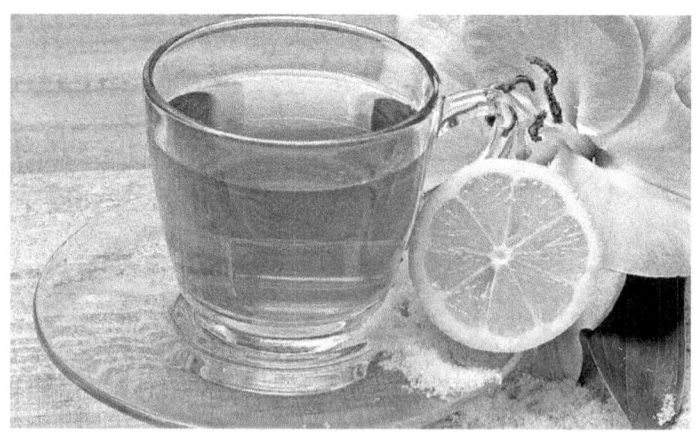

Prepare by eliminating meals over the course of 2-3 days prior. Then, you can try one full day of water only. Giving yourself time to eliminate food slowly, before beginning water fast helps to ensure that you won't suffer issues of fatigue, chronic headaches, nausea, and stomach cramping. Having enough water during a water fast, or any fast, is essential; however, too much water can disrupt your body's balance of sodium and potassium. A range of 10-14 glasses of water through the course of the day is recommended. As you gain comfort with one-day water fasting, you can then begin to allow for longer stretches once or twice a month.

From the one-day water fast, take it up to days and even three if you feel the need, or are prepared to handle that. If you start to feel symptoms of fasting like hunger or dizziness, drink a glass of water and rest. Be gentle with your body. Stand up slowly from sitting or lying positions and avoid strenuous activity and exercise. Meditation and yoga, or gentle stretching will be more appropriate during a water fast.

Attempting to exceed more than 3 days of water fasting may require consultation with a doctor or professional for guidance and aid. Consider what your goals and intentions are before excessive, long-term fasting. Mineral supplements and vitamins may be required for longer-term fasts and can even be useful and helpful, in short term fasts. Some of the supplements you can consider using are not limited to the following:

- Sodium
- Potassium
- Magnesium
- Trace minerals
- Whey
- MTC oil (medium-chain triglycerides)
- Nutritional yeast
- Collagen

There are some concerns and precautions for water fasting if you have certain medical conditions or diseases. Consult a doctor or professional before fasting if you have or suffer from any of the following:

- Advanced cancer
- Eating disorders
- High doses of prescription medication
- AIDS/HIV
- Alcoholism or drug addiction
- Advanced Type II Diabetes

- <u>Advanced neurodegenerative disorders</u>

If you are pregnant, or post-partum and breastfeeding, avoid water fasting and fasting in general for the health of you and your baby.

When you begin to plan your water fasting, there are some simple steps and guidelines to help you achieve the safest and healthiest autophagy performance. These steps are a good rule of thumb for any fast in general.

Steps and Guidelines for Water Fasting:

1. Plan water fasts when you will not be working and can have relaxing, restful periods.
2. Schedule it so you can first slowly eliminate food before transitioning to water only.
3. Schedule the length of the fast and plan what day you will slowly start to reintroduce food into your system.
4. Have the first foods available on hand before you start your water fast to prevent the need to drive to any grocery stores, in case you are feeling light-headed from the fast.
5. Choose clean, pure water, or distilled water only.

6. Fill containers of water to measure out how much you will need over the length of your fast. Try diving the measured water into to daily required amounts.

7. Reintroduce food with something simple and easy. If you are on a ketosis diet, make a smoothie of leafy greens, berries, and lemon juice, or eat a few spoonsful of high-fat yogurt. Keep it simple and small in quantity.

8. Gradually increase food intake slowly over a few days, avoiding processed foods or overly rich, decadent meals.

9. During the fast, be sure to enjoy lots of rest and relaxation. Do not overexert the body.

10. If feeling hungry, craving food, or having light-headedness, drink 1-2 glasses of water and rest for a while.

Controlling the process of healing on a deep cellular level requires some thought and planning. Engaging autophagy through water fasting can be healthy when approached in a healthy manner. Be sure to ease into a fast, slowly eliminating food, and ease out of it, slowly reintroducing food.

The benefits of water fasting are that you can clean, renew, refresh and restore your body while your internal intelligence cleans, renews, refreshes, and restores on the cellular level.

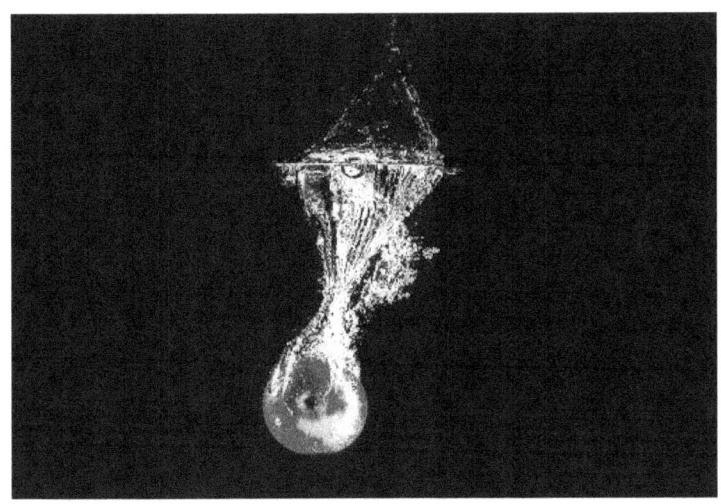

Chapter 4 Autophagy Lifestyle

Ideally, you should be aiming to fast without trying to consume any macronutrients. However, it is always good to know that there are certain macros that can start autophagy. This helps you plan your diet and fast much better.

But the question is: What macros are useful? What should you be focusing on?

Here is the first thing that you should know. If your goal is to start autophagy and when you are eating, then you should make sure that you include some form of mealtime restrictions. You can try fasting for about 20 hours, for instance, and then eat roughly 40% to 50% of the amount of energy you spend on a daily basis.

When you are taking in macros, you should ensure that they follow the guidelines below:

- Low in carbohydrates

- Have medium protein content

So, ideally, your food should have these ratios:

- 10% carbs

- 20% protein

- 25% to 30% fat

- 50% caloric deficit

This ensures that you have the right amount of macros available to you, and you do not have to stop the autophagy process at any point in time. At the same time, you are taking in low carbs.

Though whenever I mention low carbs to people, one of the common questions that I get asked is: What is the difference between a low-carb and a keto diet?

One may look at both forms of diet and think that they are both going to generate the same results. So, it does not matter if you switch one diet for the other.

The reason why people think that they are the same is that both low-carb and keto diets are aimed at reducing and, in some cases, removing the body's dependency on carbohydrates. When examined closely, you may spot differences, especially in the way that they affect your health.

To understand what we mean by that, let us try to look at each form of diet.

Low-Carb Diet

Here is a surprising fact. According to Government Dietary Guidelines for Americans, carbohydrates take up to 65% of your daily food intake.

That is a big percentage. And not a good one.

Here is another fact: There are no guidelines to tell you exactly what the low-carb diet means. There are no measurements to quantify the number of carbohydrates that make up this plan. In truth, we have noticed how this provides an excuse for manufacturers to add the term "low carb" on their labels. In the same way, a low-carb diet can mean anything. Someone can tell you that they have the best recommendations for a low-carb diet, and you may not be able to say anything against it because it might very well be true.

Keto Diet

While the rules of a low-carb diet are not exactly concrete, the keto diet works with some rules on how you approach your low-carb situation.

In order for you to go into a ketosis state, you need to make sure that you have a calorie count of fewer than 50 grams a day. By letting you know just how much calories you can consume, you are given a guideline. You can understand what you can include in your diet and what you should avoid.

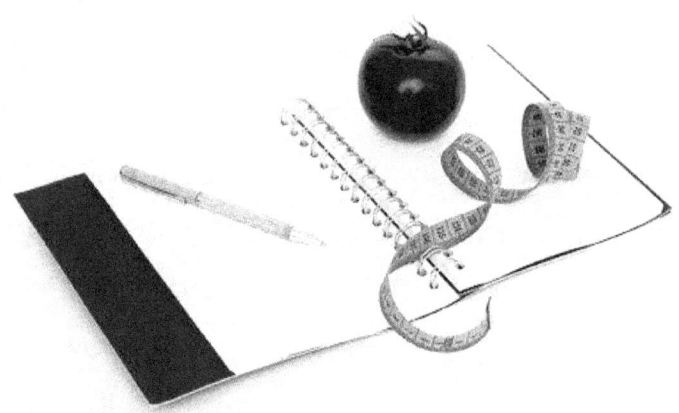

However, when you have a certain number to aim for, you can then use that as a benchmark to decide on what you are going to eat. With that, you can make sure that you are consuming the right amount of nutrients from the right source. A keto diet can make it easier for you to focus on losing weight while keeping you full.

- Ketosis may provide your body with protection against neurodegenerative diseases. But here is the kicker: it gives you long-term protection against such diseases. This is not something you can gain from a low-carb diet. One of the reasons why the keto diet was created was so that it could help people with epilepsy avid periods of seizures. In fact, for many years, neurologists have shown that the keto diet has been effective in people who are resistant to drugs that reduce epilepsy.

- Ketones are also known to act as antioxidants. This helps your brain shield itself from oxidative stress and from damages caused by stress.

When you combine the process of ketosis with autophagy, then we are looking at a host of benefits that help you live a long life that is devoid of numerous health complications.

So now that we have understood just how a keto diet is useful, what exactly are the various fasting types that we can make use of to activate ketosis and autophagy?

Let me help you with that.

Sure, those fasting techniques are some of the most popular ones, but in order to activate ketosis and take full advantage of autophagy, here are the techniques that you should be following:

OMAD (One Meal a Day)

A time-restricted feeding basically means that you are going to eat during a specific period of the day. During the remaining hours, you are going to fast. OMAD is a type of fasting that focuses on time-restricted eating. OMAD simply means "One Meal a Day" and the name says it all; you are going to have just one meal a day. One really healthy, filling and delicious meal a day.

The name does sound rather exotic. But it is a rather simple process that forces you in an OMAD plan, you follow a 23/1 fasting routine. You fast for 23 hours and then you have 1 hour to eat your food.

Alternatively, it can also be a 22/2 fasting routine. Here, you fast for 22 hours and then you take 2 hours to slowly eat your food.

But back to OMAD. Typically, people wait until dinnertime to break their fast. They use one of the many keto recipes to prepare a filling and healthy meal for themselves. The end result is that OMAD is an extreme way of doing intermittent fasting.

Protein Fasting

When you think about it, fasting is simply a pattern of eating.

You hold out on eating throughout the day and keep one time (or a few specific times, depending on what kind of fast you are holding) to have a meal that is filled with a certain type of substance (example: fat, proteins, etc.)

In many fasting techniques, people use only water. In other techniques, people use a combination of water and other liquids. Each fasting method of fasting serves a purpose and it is up to the individual to gauge what is right for them.

In the case of Protein Fasting, people withhold the consumption of protein. They fill up on other forms of nutrients such as carbs and fat (in controlled measures).

In Protein Fasting, people reduce the consumption of protein to 20 grams in one day of the week. The idea behind protein fast is to encourage the occurrence of autophagy in the body. Additionally, this type of fasting helps you burn fat without turning to OMAD or other forms of fasting.

It should be understood that if you are adopting protein fasting, then the process of autophagy takes a longer time to show its results as compared to OMAD.

With OMAD, you are going to see the results quickly, as you are expunging all unnecessary compounds from your diet for most of the day. Even when you eat, you are eating a controlled diet that consists of high fats and low carbs.

Alternate-Day Fasting

Alternate-Day Fasting or ADF (we do love our acronyms) is another form of intermittent fasting.

The foundation of this fasting is based on the idea that you fast on one day, then you eat what you feel like on the next day. Basically, it is a way to halve what you eat on a daily basis.

On the days that you are fasting, you are allowed to have calorie-free beverages. Because Alternate-Day Fasting does not entirely cut your supply of food, many people find it easier to work with than other forms of fasting.

Water Fasting

Water fasting is a fairly common practice of fasting. In fact, it has been present throughout history in some form or another.

When you are ready to do an extended water fast, one of the things you should remember is to practice with other fasting types before you try on the water fast.

Which is why I recommend that you begin with an OMAD fast. Keep the fast going on for about 2 – 3 weeks before you begin to try out extended water fast.

Another thing to remember is that you need to take it easy on yourself before you begin the fast. This means that you should not subject yourself to stressful situations. One of the ways to do that is by making sure that you are not going to your job when you are fasting. You should ideally focus on taking a couple of days off for yourself (if you can) or perhaps try out your fast during your vacation.

Another factor that you should focus on is your breathing. When you take short breaths, then your body engages in a flight or fight response. Your brain thinks that you are about to experience something dangerous. This is why most breathing exercises involve slow deep breaths. Practice breathing slowly so that you train your body to not enter into a flight or fight condition. This could cause stress to your body, which eventually leads to the consumption of more energy. This means you get hungry really fast.

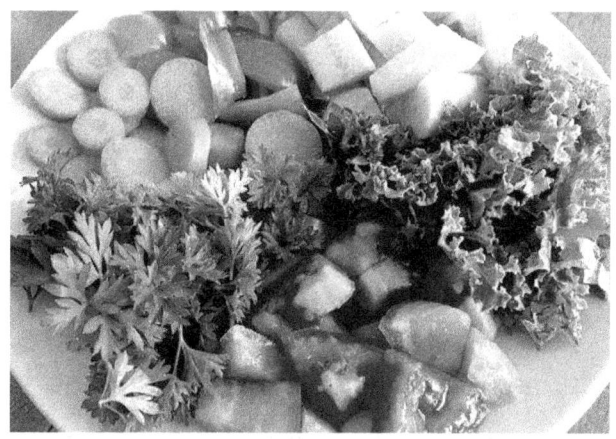

When you are ready, you need to go on extended water fast for at least 2 – 3 days.

During the fast itself, you are supposed to take in as many essential minerals as possible. For this reason, stick to mineral water. Ensure that you hydrate yourself in the morning so that you can fill up the electrolytes in your system. One of the best ways to go through with this diet is to have positive people around you. They motivate you and make you feel good about your fast. This, in turn, has positive effects on the body and the mind. You feel less stressed. You feel more motivated. More importantly, you feel happy. After all, you shouldn't be depressed about fasting!

72-Hour Fasting

I love science.

Okay, perhaps I should explain that before I go any further.

You see, I believe in the power of science to back up the tons of research conducted on intermittent fasting and autophagy. I love how we can explain what is happening on a detailed basis if we want to. Moreover, I like how we can break down the science to make it understandable for everyone.

So, why am I talking about science and putting it under a positive light? No, I did not have a sudden epiphany.

The reason why I brought up science is that most people find it difficult to believe that 72-hour fasting can be beneficial to them. They are under the impression that no one can do it. However, they forget the resiliency of the human body.

We are able to adapt to anything and one of the ways we can show that is by controlling our mindset about eating. You see, eating is something we do on a daily basis. It is not easy to give up on the habits that we are depending on sustaining us.

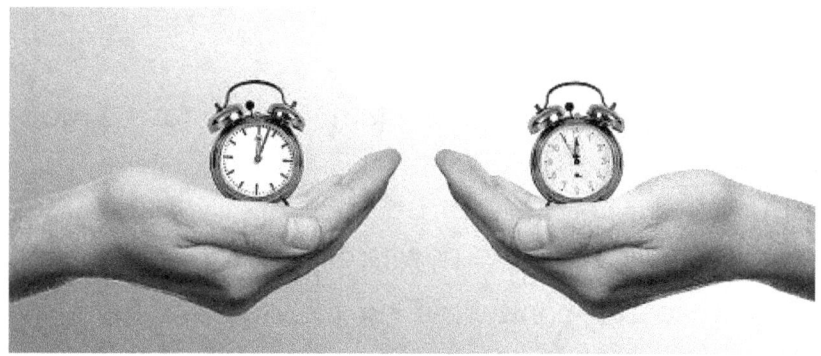

According to research conducted at the University of Southern California, abstaining from having food for even two days can result in regenerative properties for the immune system and help the body fight infections better.

The investigation took place on two- and four-day fasting

on humans (not mice this time), and the results showed that not only does the immune system get stronger, but the body gets rid of damaged parts better.

That is the benefit of going on a 72-hour fast.

When you are under this fast, you have to make sure that you understand what you can consume and what you cannot. For example, coffee and liquids such as Apple Cider Vinegar are known to curb hunger. However, you cannot just take any coffee. You are only allowed to consume plain coffee. No cream or sugar. So, say goodbye to the double espresso chocolate cream caramel Frappuccino.

One of the questions people ask about this fasting is why it is necessary when we already have a 12-hour is fasting. For one, your body is digesting food 12 hours after you have consumed it. So, biologically speaking, you haven't yet entered into a state of fasting yet.

That is why, when you are on a 72-hour fast, you make sure that you let your body complete its digestion process and get rid of the last remains of the food in your body.

One your body has completed digesting everything, you let it fast for a prolonged period of time.

However, remember that you cannot simply enter into 72-hour fasting.

You have to begin with OMAD fasting and keep at it for at least 2 to 3 weeks. Once your body gets used to OMAD fasting, then you are ready to take it to the next step.

I would also recommend that you get comfortable with water fasting for 24 hours. This will help your body prepare itself for longer fasting periods. You will have a better time getting comfortable with the 72-hour fast and you are less likely to suffer hunger pangs.

Of course, the big question is what you can and cannot drink while fasting. Apart from water fasting (where you have to focus on taking in mainly mineral water), here are some of the liquid that you can consume (no matter what fasting you have decided to adopt).

Chapter 5 Stimulating Autophagy by Mimicking Fasting

Imitating fasting with the so-called Fasting Mimicking Diet is an option for men and women who would like the benefits of fasting but may have reasons why fasting is not the best choice for them. Fasting is regarded as the gold standard in terms of stimulating autophagy because of its demonstrated use in triggering the body to remove damaged, poorly functioning, or dysfunctional components, such as cancer cells. But autophagy can also be stimulated well by diet and exercise, and in the case of the Fasting Mimicking Diet, the goal is to create a diet that resembles fasting without actually being fasting.

Recall that the idea behind fasting is that it replicates how our human ancestors would have eaten tens of thousands of years ago. At this time, human beings would have lived primarily as hunter-gatherers and not in the settled agricultural societies that characterize the way nearly all humans on Earth live today. This means that humans would not have had access to storehouses filled with grain, sugar cane, processed foods, and all the other goodies that many people take for granted today. If you wanted to eat, you would have had to hunt or fish your quarry or risk starvation.

Now, this type of life may seem harsh, but our bodies adapted to survive in this type of environmental context. It is not too different from how apex predators like lions and tigers live in their environments today. They spend much of their day sleeping or guarding their territory (essentially a fasting period), while they devote a portion of their day to hunting and eating. Naturally, when a lion hunts, he's or she is generally obeying both a predatory urge and a physical urge. He or she is hungry. This means that the fasting period actually serves to motivate the lion to hunt and hunt well. You rarely see obese or out of shape lions because their way of life demands that they are a well-oiled machine.

Well, human beings were once not too different from these apex predators. We also used to spend much of our days sleeping or guarding are territories, and we would have hunted on an empty stomach. Obesity would have been rare in social groups where food was not instantly available, and men and women would have had to hunt for survival. Today, we are constantly exposed to food in frankly enormous quantities, including high concentrations of sugar that would have baffled our ancestors. What some diets do is focus on what we take into our body as a way of preventing the lowered metabolism and energy drain that comes from eating diets high in carbohydrates.

The Fasting Mimicking Diet allows men and women who are interested in reaping the benefits of diets like the Ketogenic diet or intermittent fasting to tap into those benefits without all of the restrictions. The Fasting Mimicking Diet involves devoting five days out of a 30-day period to caloric restriction similar to what is seen in Keto while the remaining 25 days are less restrictive. The idea here is to place the body in something akin to ketosis in order to mobilize adipose (fat) stores for energy rather than the circulating blood sugars that most people who eat sugar and carbs constantly use for energy. This excess sugar is not only used for energy but stored as fat which is counterproductive and leads to obesity. By cutting out sugar sources, you force your body to look to other more natural energy sources. This leads to benefits like fat mobilization (lipolysis) through autophagy as well as other benefits like improved insulin sensitivity.

Basics of the Fasting Mimicking Diet

The essential fact to remember about the Fasting Mimicking Diet is that during your five days of the fasting-mimicking you are drastically reducing your caloric intake but not actually going on a fast. A fast means that you are not taking in any calories at all, and during your fasting-mimicking days, you would be taking in perhaps as little as 500 calories. Five hundred calories would be equivalent to one large cheeseburger at a fast-food restaurant or a large highly processed pastry (that is high in fat and carbohydrates).

As the Ketogenic diet, what you eat during your fasting-mimicking days is important as the idea is to trick your body into thinking that you are fasting. You do this by eating a diet that is relatively low in carbohydrates, but not as low as it would be in Keto. Recall that the hallmark

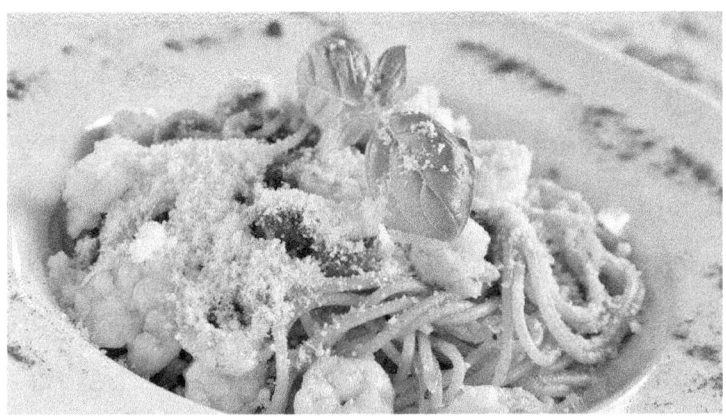

of Keto is that carb intake is reduced to almost zero. In Fasting Mimicking, you may take in about 30% of your calories from carbohydrates. It is okay to do this because your total caloric intake is so low (between 500 to 1000 calories for five days).

The idea here is that this period of low calories is recognized by the body as starvation, which is the essential goal of a fast. Fasting and starvation are distinguished by the body merely by duration. For example, any period of no food is technical "starvation" to the body although we tend to use this term only to refer to periods where individuals have no caloric intake for a prolonged period usually due to circumstances outside of their control. Prolonged starvation can lead to syndromes like kwashiorkor or marasmus that are seen in countries experiencing drought or other calamities.

To return to our main point: tricking your body into thinking that it is in starvation because of days of low calories triggers autophagy. Most people on the Fasting Mimicking Diet do it because they want to lose weight, but all of the other benefits of autophagy can be reaped here, too. This is a recurring theme in this book. Autophagy confers a host of benefits to the person who stimulates it, and you might find that you reap positive health advantages that you had not anticipated, like a sense of energy and well-being.

The main benefit of the Fasting Mimicking Diet is that you can enter something like a fast without some of the downsides of a fast (or starvation). Some people may find fasting difficult because they have never done it before. Others may have health concerns that render fasting inadvisable. The Fasting Mimicking Diet allows you to stimulate autophagy similar to how you would in a fast. Again, research suggests that fasting of 18 to 24 hours is the best way to stimulate autophagy (and reap its benefits), but not everyone can do this. Some people use the Fasting Mimicking Diet as a starting point to attempting fasting in the future.

Example of a Fasting Mimicking Diet Protocol

A typical Fasting Mimicking Diet protocol consists of 5 consecutive days of fasting-mimicking followed by 25 days without fasting mimicking. Most practitioners of this diet carefully follow their macronutrients (macros) just as they would in the Ketogenic diet. Typically, the first of the five days is lower on carbohydrates, but the carbs are increased slightly in the following days. There are different ways to go about this diet, but an example of a diet using this protocol is shown below. The percentage shown is the relative percentage of total calories for the day from that macronutrient. Recall that the three main macronutrients are fat, protein, and carbohydrates.

First Day (Day 1):

A total of five to six calories total for each pound of body weight, so about 800 calories for a 160-pound person

Fat: 60%

Protein: 10%

Carbohydrate: 30%

Following Days (Days 2 through 5):

A total of three to four calories in total for each pound of body weight, so about 480 calories for a 160-pound person

Fat: 50%

Protein: 10%

Carbohydrate: 40%

Tips to Help with Fasting

Some people learn best with tips. Let's face it, there is a lot to learn about autophagy, and no one is expected to be an expert after reading about the subject for an hour or two. You will learn the most about this process after you have given stimulating it a try. Tips can help you whether your goal is to lose weight or too fast for days and days in order to kill cancer cells in your body. Here are some tips to help get you started.

Tip 1. You do not have to skip meals in order to fast.

Although fasting means that you are not eating, it does not necessarily mean that you have to skip a meal. What are we talking about here? People who intermittent fast and have a 16/8 split, for example, are still able to eat a normal (or relatively normal) three meals a day. They just have to do this in a smaller window than they normally might. So your breakfast might be at 10 AM, your lunch might be at 1:30, and your dinner might be at 5:30. Fasting is a different word from "starvation" for a reason. Fasting does not have to mean that you are miserable.

Tip 2. Having coffee before you start your fast (or something else with fat in it) can keep you satiated.

There is a lot of talk about whether or not coffee drinking should be considered breaking a fast. In truth, there are some calories in coffee, but they are so low (generally less than 100 calories) that they are not counted by many people who fast. But for the purpose of this trip, we are thinking about ways that you can work coffee in before you fast. If you have coffee right before a fast it can help keep you satiated, especially if it contains some cream or other additives with a little added fat in it.

Tip 3. Drinking water during your fast can help you feel fuller.

Water fasting is a thing for a reason. No, not because some people are lunatics who like to drink water until it makes them sick (which is actually a thing). Water can help you feel fuller. There is some debate as to whether this is due to receptors in your stomach being stretched by the volume of water or because of some other reason, but all you need to know is that works. It may not be a good idea to replace all of your next five meals with water when you are just starting out with this, but it is something to keep in mind. Having a tall glass of water can help you stave off your hunger when your goal is to fast for a short while longer.

Tip 4. Work your way up to longer fasts rather than jumping into a long fast early on.

Taking baby steps is always a good idea. When it comes to fasting, this means not jumping into a highly restrictive fast, but working your way up to it. It is not difficult to do. Indeed, some people do this by first engaging in an autophagy diet like intermittent fasting and then working their way up to a whole day fast or longer. Again, you always have the option of drinking water as part of your fast thereby incorporating a water fasting diet. Most people who fast for days and days started out where you might be now - a little overweight and wondering if it is possible to make a major change in their life. The answer is "yes," it is possible.

Tip 5. Eating a pinch of salt during a fast can quench your hunger pangs.

Some fasting experts recommend eating a pinch of salt during periods when you are tempted to break your fast.

Salt is sodium chloride, which means it contains two ions that are essential in your body's homeostasis. Sodium chloride not only can satiate your taste buds, but it can help you feel fuller (and better) by keeping the water in your body. Have you noticed that when you drink large quantities of water you tend to urinate it out relatively quickly? That is because your body needs sodium chloride in order to keep the water in your body's cells and tissues. So, here is a little trick. If you are having problems with your fast, try adding a pinch of salt.

Tip 6. Apple cider vinegar may break your fast, but it will help you while intermittent fasting.

Apple cider vinegar contains acetic acid which assists in vitamin and mineral uptake in the body. Apple cider vinegar also contains polyphenols that boost the immune system.

It is a matter of debate whether or not apple cider vinegar will break a fast. Some in the health industry argue that it does not contain enough calories to impact insulin so it will not break a fast. Others say that apple cider vinegar is not zero calories, and even one calorie is enough to break a fast. Even if you drink this right before you start a fast you can have a benefit during your fast. To incorporate this type of vinegar into your fasting regimen. You will not regret it.

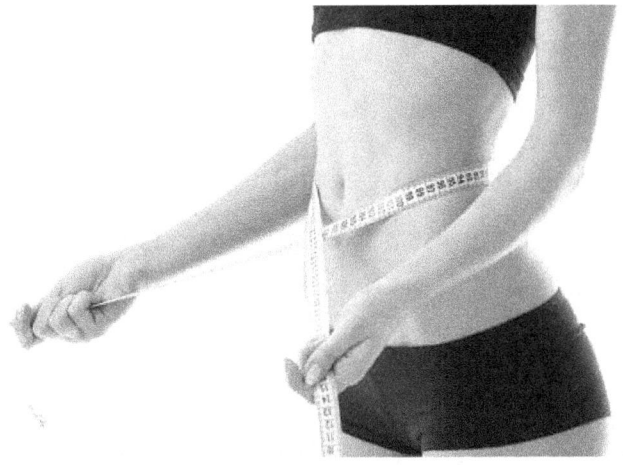

Tip 7. Adding a pinch of sea salt to your water can help you maintain your fast.

Salt does not have to be a bad thing. We have already spoken about adding a pinch of salt, but it is important here to talk about the benefits of all-natural options during your fast. Processed products, like artificial sweeteners, can actually cause problems with your fast because they can derail your metabolism. Even salt can have other things added to it that make it more than just regular salt. So if you are planning to use salt to help you along in your fast, try sea salt or another of nature's varieties of this substance.

Tip 8. Avoid supplements like branched-chain amino acids during your fast because these will cause an insulin spike.

Whether or not to take supplements is always a big question when it comes to fast. Many people continue to take supplements during their fast without being aware that they are technically breaking their fast because their supplements are not calorie-free. Even branched-chain amino acids (or BCAAS) contain calories, which makes sense considering that some people actually use these for energy during a workout. So here is a tip: it is okay to take supplements and vitamins before or after a fast, but they should generally be avoided during your fasting window. If you do not, then you really are not fasting.

Tip 9. Do not add creams or sweeteners to drinks you are consuming during your fast (such as coffee); you also should not use artificial sweeteners like those contained in diet sodas.

Tip 10. Tea will not break a fast so drink lots of green tea (which will cause you to feel satiated).

Tea is another one of those products that have tons of questions surrounding it when it comes to fasting. Does tea break your fast? Although some choose to avoid tea and anything else substantive like this during a fast, many fitness experts argue that tea will not break your fast. They argue this because tea does not contain compounds that impact metabolism (specifically, it does not impact insulin causing an insulin spike) so you can drink as much tea as you like, and your body will still think you are fasting. Green tea can also help you to feel satiated while you are on your fast

Chapter 6 Tips to Control Hunger

Even though the metabolic state of ketosis has proven to have some hunger reducing benefits, you might still struggle with hunger urges in the beginning stages of your diet. These are common and expected – especially if you snack avidly before starting the diet.

But there are ways to control your hunger, and you really can be stronger than the voice inside your head telling you to eat that last piece of chocolate cake – do not do it.

Make sure that you eat enough protein. When you have enough protein in your diet, you will not feel the need to eat as much as proteins promote feelings of fullness.

A fiber-rich diet will also aid in warding off those hunger pains as the fibers will release hormones indicating you are full.

Solid foods will leave you feeling fuller over a liquid metal. So, you might want to eat that breakfast of eggs and bacon over the strawberry smoothie the next time you have a busy day.

Decaf coffee can help reduce your appetite. Studies have shown that decaf coffee can repress appetite cravings for up to three hours after it has been consumed. And since decaf coffee is on the approved list of keto beverages, drink away!

Fill up on water before meals. This way you will also eat less and feel fuller for a longer period of time. When you drink enough water to stretch the stomach, this will signal to the brain that you are full. In a way, you are tricking your brain into believing that it has received the food it is asking for.

Change the plates you eat on. When you eat from smaller plates, you will feel full just the same as if your plate and portion was larger. In this way, you can lessen your food intake and not feel deprived of it.

Get enough sleep! The more rested you feel, the fewer cravings you will have. Sounds odd? Well, studies have proven that a person who is rested indicates a higher level of fullness after they ate the same breakfast as those who did not sleep well.

If you are in a stressful environment, try to find a way to reduce or eliminate the stress. Stress is directly related to a person feeling like they need to eat more food as it can be a coping mechanism. Try a stress ball if you cannot reduce the stress in your environment.

How To Keto At A Restaurant

Just because you are on the keto diet does not mean you cannot go out and enjoy it! Just make sure you are aware of what you can and cannot eat while you are out, and resist giving in to temptations.

Luckily for those on the keto diet, you can find something keto-friendly on almost any restaurant menu!

Going to a burger joint? Just skip the bun! Avoid the carbs and enjoy the burger with all the vegetables that would normally come with it. Get a side salad or side of pickles instead of those French fries, and you are good to go!

For breakfast your options are wide. You can eat all the eggs you want, add some bacon or sausage and cheese and you are good to go. Just remember to skip the regular coffee and go for decaf. Also, no bread or biscuits.

Eat all the barbecue you want! Just ask them to hold the sauce. Pulled pork, brisket, and ribs? Yummy! And all the things you can eat.

You are bound to find a bowl of yummy leafy greens in there somewhere.

Going to a restaurant that gives you complimentary chips and salsa? Or even bread? Let the server know beforehand not to bring it to the table. If it is out of sight, odds are you will not even miss it.

Oops! I Ate Something I Should Not Have

Okay, so you messed up. Now what? Well, the answer to that is actually very simple.

First, establish why you cheated. Was it a social gathering you were too tempted to say no to? A special holiday? Or are you still experience cravings.

While it can take the body 3-6 weeks to get fully adapted to being in a state of ketosis, you might want to double-check your macronutrients if you are constantly craving food and ensure you are getting all the nutrients you need.

When you cheat on your keto diet the stage of ketosis, you are in can depend on your reaction. If you are at the beginning of ketosis, it might be a bigger setback than if you were fat adapted (this means your body is now adapted to using fat as a fuel source).

The first thing that cheating might do is raise your blood sugar levels. Be wary that if you cheat once, you should not do it again as it can be harder each time to get your body back to the metabolic state of ketosis.

You might also experience a sugar rush and sugar crash if you cheated with something high in sugar. With your body not being used to that amount of sugar, it can cause an imbalance. It might be tempting to continue to give in to the sugar cravings once they have started, but it is important to remain strong against them.

Cheating on your keto diet – especially if you have been an avid keto follower for a while – can have many adverse reactions as your body will not be used to processing all those carbs and sugars. Remember, keto is not just a diet but also a lifestyle choice and change.

If you want to limit your reaction to your cheat day and stay ahead and in ketosis, autophagy will become your best friend. Paired with going back to your keto routine, autophagy will also help prompt your body to keep its blood ketone levels elevated. When autophagy, you can choose which way works best for you, you might find that skipping your next meal is the answer.

Drinking lots of water will also help you deal with the symptoms. Drinking water will make you feel full, and therefore you will be less likely to give in into any

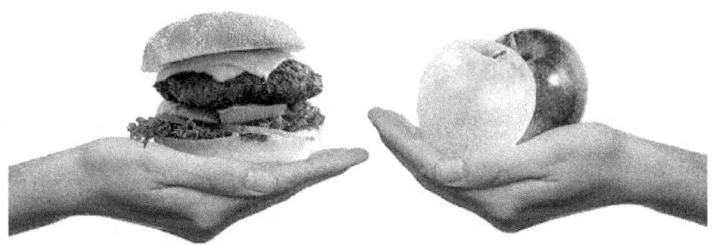

additional cravings.

If you are hungry, stay away from the sugar and go toward your healthy fats! These will fill you up, and they follow your keto diet guidelines.

To stay away from the monotony of the keto diet, switch it up. There are thousands of recipes out there for you to try and keep your palate invested in your lifestyle. Go through the end of this book and see if there is not a recipe you have not tried yet! Variety is life!

If you are really struggling with the symptoms from your cheat day, take a shortcut. Find those exogenous ketones and take them. They can help you get back on track fast, as long as you are following the keto diet after your cheat. The supplements do not work with a high carb diet.

Key Points

Maintaining the keto lifestyle is not always easy, and you are bound to have a slip up now and then – especially in the beginning. Do not be too hard on yourself, you are your own biggest critic. Take a deep breath and just focus.

· Make sure your goals are attainable.

· Do not rely only on your own determination to manage to keto lifestyle change, implement other changes to ensure you follow through.

· There are several ways to curb your appetite if you are still experiencing cravings – drinking lots of water is only one of them.

· A majority of restaurants will have something you can eat while on keto, so don't be shy to go out!

· If you slip up, don't be too hard on yourself. There are lots of ways to get yourself back on the keto slide.

As more studies about the keto diet are being done, the

list of benefits keeps growing. It might seem hard to keep up, so let us go over them so you can make an informed decision about what your personal goals are with keto!

Why Is The Keto Diet Special?

The keto diet has many benefits that most mainstream diets do not have. There are several reasons why the keto diet is better than most other low carb diets. The main one is sustainability. The Keto diet does call for a drastic change in the way you eat, but it also promotes a healthier eating lifestyle.

The keto diet is different from other diets because it calls for a limited amount of proteins to be consumed, a drastic reduction in carbohydrate intake, and high-fat consumption. Even though the keto diet calls for high-fat consumption, the emphasis here is on healthy, unprocessed fats.

In our daily diets we might still eat a lot of fat with the normal carbohydrates we take in, but most of these fats will be over-processed and unhealthy for us. The keto diet focuses on healthy whole fatty foods.

The cutting of carbs means a more consistent stream of energy. Since carbs are sugars once we consume them, they can cause sugar highs and crashes. Eliminating these and entering the metabolic state of ketosis we are ensuring the likelihood that our energy levels stay the same and do not dip and dive.

Studies have also proven that the keto diet has proven longer-term results with consistent weight loss, far more than a low-fat diet.

Evidence has also shown that over time the keto diet has helped manage certain diseases and disorders.

Remember, the keto diet was once used as a therapy. One of the major benefits that put this diet a cut above the rest is its success in minimizing the seizures experienced by those with epilepsy. Particularly in children with epilepsy. The main group this diet has benefited are children who suffer from focal seizures. Have you ever heard of another diet whose benefits included being used as a therapy for seizures?

The Keto diet not only shows promise in reducing seizures, but it also has shown results for women with polycystic ovarian syndrome (PCOS). It has been proven that high carbohydrate diets negatively affect women with PCOS. A pilot study was conducted using five women that were watched over a twenty-four week period. The study concluded that the keto diet increased weight loss, aided hormone balance, improved hormone ratios, and improved fasting insulin. While more research is still needed, and additional experiments will need to be conducted to confirm all the results found in the preliminary study; those are still fabulous results for women with PCOS on the keto diet.

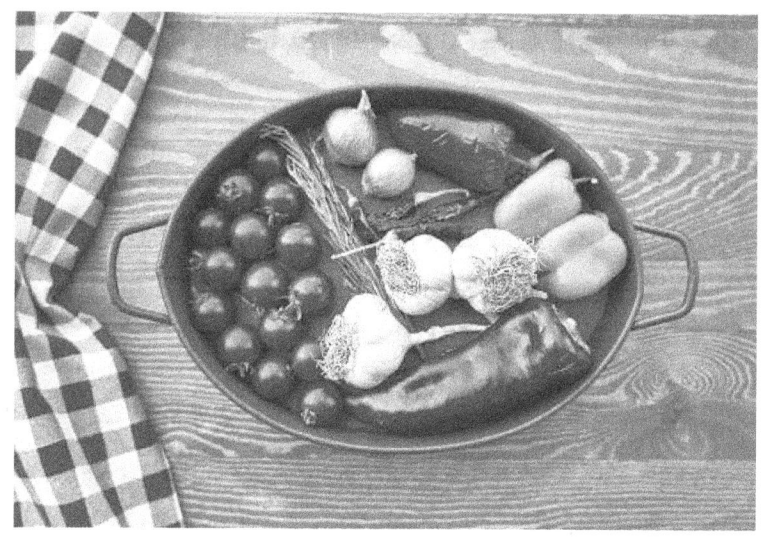

The keto diet relies on the use of your ketone molecules for fuel. These ketones are good for your brain's function. There is evidence that they even help with memory loss patients. Because of the change from carbs to ketones, your body will also have hormone hunger changes. That's another benefit that the keto diet brings to the table that other diets fail to provide without supplements! You will likely feel fewer hunger cravings on the keto diet, and you will find yourself snacking less than you did before you were on the diet.

The keto diet also reduces acne! Yes, you read that right. Because most of our daily diets consist of refined and processed carbohydrates, our faces can tend to break out more. But on the keto diet, those kinds of carbs are not allowed to be consumed. The result is that without those unhealthy carbs, our skin clears up. Acne has a direct correlation with our diets and what we put into our bodies.

Keto is good for your heart! Studies have shown that while on the keto diet, the heart health of individuals went up. This is due to the fact that those who were on the keto diet were reported to have higher levels of good cholesterol (HDL), and their bad cholesterol (LDL) levels went down significantly.

While other diets might help you lose weight, they are mostly for the short-term and not the long-term benefits.

Besides weight loss, ketogenic diets help with overall body function and health! Research has shown time and time again that the keto diet has an overall positive impact on certain disorders and diseases.

Who Should Not Be on Keto

While the keto diet is awesome! And it does help with weight loss and a healthier lifestyle; there are some conditions that would mean you should not partake in the keto diet.

Anyone who has kidney damage should not be on the keto diet. Similarly, women who are pregnant or breastfeeding should not use keto diet methods. If you have type 1 diabetes, the keto diet could have some adverse effects on you due to the risk of hypoglycemia (low blood sugar.) The diet is also not recommended for those without gallbladders as it is a diet high in fat content.

The keto diet requires you to make a complete overhaul of the way you eat. Most diets will tell you to reduce the intake of fat and eat more carbohydrates. Keto is different in that it requires almost no carbohydrates and all the good healthy high fats you want – sort of, within reason. And, as with any drastic change, consult your doctor before starting the keto diet to ensure it is a fit for you.

Just a few takeaways about why the keto diet rocks!

· It helps with short-term and long-term weight loss.

· It can help you manage or minimize the risks of other types of diseases and conditions.

· It leads to healthier eating habits.

· It promotes eating whole foods over processed foods.

· Always consult your doctor before making a drastic lifestyle change.

Chapter 7 The Importance of Staying Hydrated

The importance of water in the body cannot be overemphasized. Even when you are not fasting, it is critical to do all in your capacity to stay hydrated, let alone when you are staying away from food. The body is made up of many organs, and to keep up with their functions, they must be hydrated. There is no specific amount of water to drink while on the fast.

However, we advise you to take a cue from your urine to give an insight into how hydrated your body is. Pale yellow urine is what you should be after. Dark yellow urine, on the other hand, is a sure sign of dehydration. Not drinking enough water could make the fast pretty tricky. It sets the pace for fatigue, headache, lightheadedness, and many other complications.

Besides helping the body keep up with its function, staying hydrated helps curb the severity of hunger pangs. And to make things interesting, you can add cucumber slices, mint, fruit or a squeeze of lemon, etc. to your water

What are the best ways to stay hydrated while having an intermittent fast or keto diet?

Stay Away from Sugar Foods and Drinks

Processed sugary drinks and food, spicy foods, etc. should be avoided while breaking your fast. Even though this might temporarily quench your thirst, it rewards you with an instant spike in blood sugar level. This spike later causes a crash and triggers dehydration. Even when cooking, resist using excess spice and salt.

Excess salt is harmful to the body and is present in many food items. Besides minimizing processed foods, we recommend switching to healthy salt types like Himalayan salt or Celtic salt.

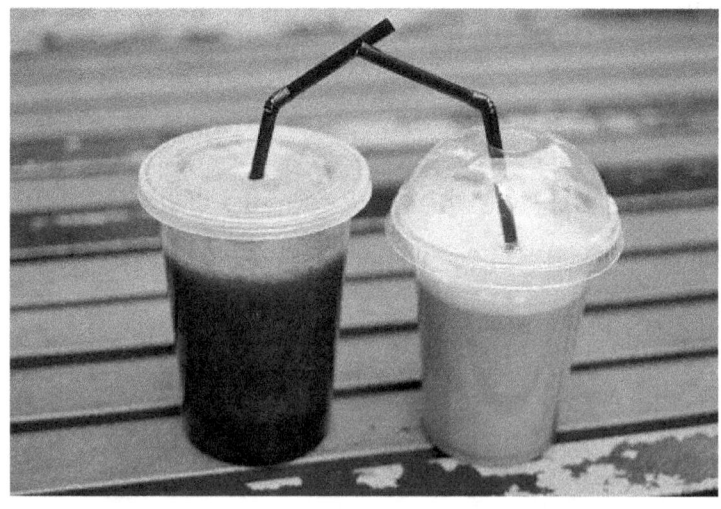

Spread Your Water Intake

Intermittent fasting and the keto diet is not a do or die. You are only restricting calories, not water. As a result, you are free to drink water, in whatever quantity, whenever you want. With this in mind, be sure to spread your water intake throughout your fast, especially if you are going with protracted fast.

Be sure to have a bottle of water handy, especially in the hot afternoon, to quench your thirst when the pangs get tough.

Consume more Fruits and Vegetables

Without a doubt, this has to do with fruits and vegetables low in carbs and sugar. There are some fruits and vegetables that are high in water content. They can help keep you hydrated and nourished after fasting.

We recommend fruits like tomatoes, vegetables, celery, and watermelons. Being high in water content, they can keep you hydrated. Vegetables are useful salad components if you can't eat them raw. There are fruits high in fiber as well, which can help you stay full for long periods, in addition to vital minerals essential for optimum function of your body and strength for the fast.

Limit Exposure to Heat

We understand you might not be able to control this, especially if you have to work in the sun. This is why you have to be strategic with the fast. Schedule your fast to time when you will neither expend too much energy nor be required to be in the sun.

As much as you can, avoid heat. Hot temperatures raise the temperature of your body, which triggers sweating, causing loss of body fluid, something you want to avoid. Wear comfortable clothes, limit time outdoors, and stick to cool environments.

Chia Water

You can employ the power of chia seeds in staying hydrated while fasting. They are high in fiber (which will keep you full), protein, and calcium. Being high in antioxidants, they draw in water, keeping you full longer. Since chia seeds expand when exposed to water, it gets thicker; so, we recommend drinking it with a straw.

One tablespoon of chia seeds in half a liter of water is all you need. You are not mandated to use this ratio strictly anyway, and you can tweak it to your taste. Leave the mixture for about 15 minutes to get a paste-like texture. You can use mint-infused water if you like some flavor.

Be Smart with Caffeine

We know you love tea and coffee, but they contain caffeine. While we have nothing against caffeine, it has a diuretic effect which fosters urine production. This flushes a lot of water out of your body, leaving you dehydrated.

When you have excessive caffeine, you end up losing water, which is not what you want. With this in mind, we recommend staying away from caffeine for the period of your fast. Stick with water and spice it up with the ingredients recommended above, if you like.

Effective Methods to Control Hunger While Fasting

When intermittent fasting for autophagy or trying out the keto diet, one of the greatest challenges is keeping hunger in check. The concept of intermittent fasting is like eating restrictions in which you eat all your meals within a specific window. During the period while you go without food, your body taps energy from stored fats and uses it for power.

It is, therefore, not uncommon for people to deal with

dizziness, headaches, and loss of energy at the onset of the fast, which could be downright discouraging. This is your body crying against the sudden discomfort the lack of food has caused. The good news, however, is that the body will get accustomed to it, with time. This is why we dedicated this section to guide you on how to go about handling the annoying hunger pangs that come at you with full force.

It is, however, vital that we sound a note of warning here. Be sure to contact your doctor before commencing intermittent fasting.

Apple Cider Vinegar

There are tremendous health benefits to apple cider vinegar. Besides helping with digestion and weight loss, it can keep you full and satisfied while fasting. We recommend drinking apple cider vinegar in the early hours of the day.

All you need is a teaspoon or two, and you can get the many benefits of apple cider vinegar.

Work on Your Mindset

At times, when intermittent fasting, it is not the fact that we did not eat that caused hunger. Instead, if you are preoccupied with thoughts of food, hunger might come knocking on you hard. The human mind is so powerful that most time when we think we are hungry; it is the thought of hunger that is making us feel hungry.

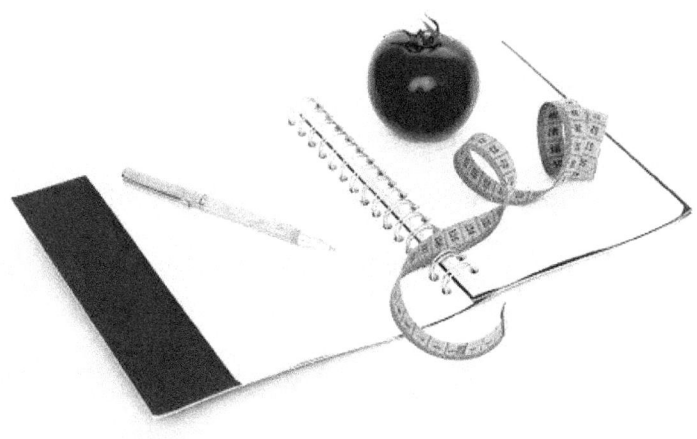

Rather than letting your thoughts dwell on the absence of food, we recommend switching your thoughts to other positive and essential things. Think about the benefits of the sacrifice you are paying. Think about the delayed aging, improved health, and cleansing going on in your body system. Reflect on the break your digestive system is having. When your thoughts dwell on these positive and important things, the feeling of hunger might be suppressed.

Concentrate on Activities You Love

If you have nothing tangible to occupy your time while on intermittent fasting, the hunger pangs will come knocking at you with full force. This is the time you can concentrate on things you love. We recommend dedicating time to watching a comedy series, writing a journal, taking an online class, and picking up a hobby. The goal is to keep your mind occupied so that it has no chance to listen to the rumblings of your tummy or even think about food.

Keep Up with Oral Hygiene

Another distraction tactic when hunger pangs come at you without mercy is to have a quick brush. It is an excellent way to curb the craving. Besides, there is something about having a fresh breath which reduces the desire to eat. With this in mind, keeping your oral hygiene in top condition is an excellent way to have a successful fast.

Reduce Demanding Tasks and Get Busy

While we are not asking you to sit around all day doing nothing, it is essential to be careful of what you engage yourself in. Any activity physically demanding can make you very hungry. This is because of the tendency of the body to release cortisol when stressed, increasing the desire to eat. In addition to going to the movies and taking up a series, we recommend going for a stroll, watching the birds, etc.

In contrast to going about demanding activity, we recommend focusing your strength on other productive aspects. Fasting is known to give improved energy and productivity. With a list of less tasking activities, you will be so distracted that you will not know when it is time to eat.

Sleep Well and Sleep Early

One of the most effective ways to curb hunger is to go to bed early. Ideally, humans need eight hours of sleep every day. Many of us, however, do not get this much sleep. Sleeping well and sleeping early is magical as it reduces the amount of time you spend in the fasted state. Take a 16:8 fasting protocol, for instance. If you spend eight hours in a bed, half of your fasting window is gone already.

Have you ever noticed that you tend to be quite hungry when you do not get enough sleep? This is because our body is trying to compensate for increased energy demand as a result of staying up. This is why a deep, long, and restorative sleep is key to helping keep the hunger pangs at bay while fasting.

Engage in a Warm Bath

Bear in mind that while fasting, you want to do anything that will take your mind away from the hunger pangs. One such thing is a warm bath. A warm bath is helpful for several reasons. First, it is a good way of taking care of yourself and instilling good habits. Also, fasting often lowers body temperature; hence, a warm bath will help raise body temperature and having a warm bath is like a distraction, especially when the hunger comes knocking at you.

Avoid Sugar Like the Plague

This does not even have to do with the fasting window. During your feasting window, we recommend concentrating on whole and healthy foods. Sugar and its many forms, alongside processed foods, are completely frowned upon. This is because the sugar will likely increase your appetite during your eating window. Avoid all forms of sugary food during your feasting window to keep from shooting yourself in the leg.

<u>Forget You Have a Kitchen</u>

Okay, we understand that you might not be able to forget that a kitchen exists in your apartment, but you can lock it up and keep the keys. You might not have to deal with cravings and hunger if you are not taking too many trips to the kitchen.

In addition to staying away from the kitchen, avoid the restaurant, grocery stores, and parties. The idea is to stay away from food as the slightest aroma or sight of food might trigger cravings. It is also a bad idea to prepare food for others. If you are a mom or a housewife with kids, schedule your fasting period when you have time to yourself. Besides, if you have an understanding partner, I see no reason why he wouldn't want to take up the responsibility of cooking!

<u>Chew Gum</u>

What if all else fails? What if you cannot resist the hunger pangs? What if the urge to eat something becomes irresistible? Chewing gum is a last resort you can take to keep your fast going, without breaking the fast. Have in mind, however, that chewing gum will only curb your cravings for a moment, but it could reward you with a horrible feeling of hunger later.

The logic is simple; you are chewing, your body systems, intestine, and all are all excited in preparation for the semi-digested food that they think is coming in soon. However, the endless waiting and waiting will lead them to revolt, making the hunger come at you fiercely. Chewing gum is best used near the end of your fasting window. Also, be sure not to chew more than two pieces of gum at a time to avoid insulin spike.

What if you get off track?

Fasting for autophagy should be seen as a tool to make life better. In other words, it is not a do or die affair. Should you get off track, it is not an avenue to get discouraged or beat yourself up. Bear in mind that you are supposed to ease into the fast. This means you go gradually, listening to your body as you progress. Any attempt to delve into it might make you crash and get you off track.

In any case, if you get off track, give yourself a day or two to get enough nutrients, and start again. Be sure to move easily this time around. Arm yourself with the tips to keep hunger in check and ease yourself gradually.

Mistakes to Avoid When Inducing Autophagy

So far, so good. We have examined the basics of autophagy and what you have to know about it. We have also shed light on the most effective ways to go about activating autophagy.

On a final note, we will be shedding light on common mistakes people make while trying to activate autophagy. Whether you want to launch it by fasting, starting the keto diet, or exercise, you have to keep these in mind to enable you to have a smooth transition to autophagy and also reap the benefits.

Using Autophagy as an Excuse to Feed on Junks

With intermittent fasting, there is a restriction in the eating window. The keto diet, on the other hand, involves being careful with the number of carbs, protein, and fats consumed.

However, the fact that you have to restrict your meals to a particular feeding interval does not mean you should not concentrate on functional foods. Bear in mind intermittent fasting places some levels of stress on the body. The body system is not getting an adequate supply of nutrients. Even with a keto diet, only some classes of food are allowed. Many people sabotage their own success by the kind of food they eat. Remember part of the reasons for autophagy is to cleanse the body of dead and useless body cells. What is the essence of this if you are going to jump right back to feeding on thrash?

Besides, it is also vital to note that processed foods should not be eaten. Junk food rewards your body system with processed fat that works against your aim of activating autophagy. Besides, even if you get to activate autophagy, you might not be so lucky to gain all the benefits associated with it.

This calls for being smart with the sort of food you feed on when breaking your fast. Since you're eating window is limited, you must be very mindful of what you eat. Besides, for those on the keto diet, there are healthy food choices that will not make you miss regular food in any way. It is essential to be careful with your food choices. Concentrate on consuming the right balance of essential macronutrients (healthy fats, lean protein, and carbs).

Also, if you will be reducing calorie intake, it is vital to concentrate only on healthy and nutritious calories. That you are restricting calories is not an excuse to focus only on substandard sources.

Restricting Calories During the Eating Window

While you are not supposed to overeat while breaking your fast, restricting calories as well is not a good idea. This is one of the most common mistakes many people fall into. Since your eating window is now limited, it is vital to get all the important macronutrients and calories in. If you eat less, you might feel less hungry, which will help you if you aim to lose weight. However, you might have to face serious hunger pangs later, as well as the effect of your body not getting enough calories.

For this reason, as you restrict calories, be sure to and eat enough healthy foods. This is, however, not an excuse to pack in thousands of calories in a single meal. While you might go with this when trying to lose weight, it is not advisable. If you want to build lean muscle, you have to eat a few extra calories to compensate for the fasting window.

With this, you get the metabolic benefits of fasting since there are new stem cells that will come in handy during the fasting window.

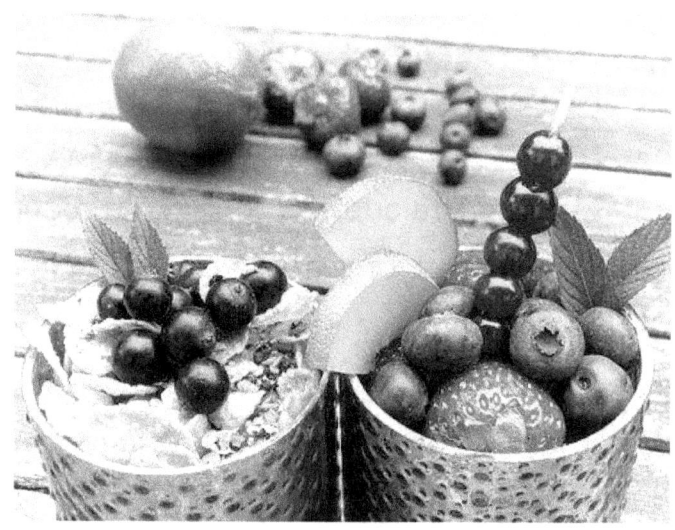

Chapter 8 Stimulating Autophagy by mimicking food

Example of a Fasting-Mimicking diet protocol

Some meat plans are offered in this scenario to make the reader know about the formation of a fast mimicking diet

Basics of the fasting-mimicking diet and its importance in lifestyle

First, let us discuss what is meant by a lifestyle? The lifestyle of an individual is based on his daily routine, his calorie intake, his daily processions, and the repute; he carries along with him while pursuing the daily lifestyle. The lifestyle of a starlet can be very famous. He will ride new vehicles; he will look healthy and try his best to do the best in his movies. He will professionalize his life by working hard and he will adopt a healthy regime in his routine to be successful. Therefore, the daily choices, in terms of food, clothing and routine procession, a lifestyle can be defined.

Now why the alkaline lifestyle is so popular? What basic ingredients, it holds in it that makes it famous. The result of having a fast mimicking diet is very successful in its reflection and the confidence that any individual can harness through it is the real reason why the intake of a fast mimicking diet can be very effective. People deem it famous because they become famous or at-least become renowned to the fact that they are in the limelight. The idea of popularity can be assessed through this notion that eating a fast mimicking diet can make you fit and being fit, can be the source of a healthy lifestyle. While having a lifestyle, you can do a lot of works, a lot of practice and can execute many frameworks through effective planning. This argument can be further prolonged to many levels of analysis.

The first level of analysis is the individualistic level. On an individualistic level, individuals get revered to be the lean and muscular figures that have the potential to succeed in life. They can do a lot of things like move composedly in their professional careers, they can be focus on their diets and prevent their bodies from being affected by many health diseases like TB, heart cancer, kidney stone and even fracture of bones. They can go to popular lifestyles like the fashion industry and even apply for acting careers. Therefore, on an individualistic level, one can easily transform the credentials of his self into a famous personality. All he needs to do is to have a fast mimicking diet in his routine.

On a social level, a society steams into the portions of activeness and recognition through a fast mimicking diet. A society is able to get all the intention and popularity if it follows a fast mimicking diet because the functions of society and the correlation of social institutions can be effective in their progress and allowing the intake of a fast mimicking diet will always open a plethora of opportunities for the society to flourish in the status-quo. Also, the norms and values are equally translated into the successful sustenance of any society and the claws of societal decadence are easily averted. So, on a societal level, there are many features of having a fast mimicking diet that can be very helpful for a society to boost its formation in the contemporary. All the societies, whether western or eastern, must be allowed to have a taste of this fast mimicking diet and this diet could be effective for the nourishment of their lifestyles.

The state-level can also be analyzed while discussing the popularity of a fast mimicking diet. The state is an engine for any country's progress and without its efficient working and statehood; a nation cannot become successful in geopolitics and geo-economics. Leaders need to adopt a fast mimicking diet system that can be healthy for their country's lead and they can steer the nation's ship with productive body metabolisms. For instance, the food regimen of China's President, Mr. Xi Jinping is of significance. The guy does not claim to have a fast mimicking diet but still, his bodily gestures coupled with prudent state policies make him be a decisive state man. Also, there are many leaders that abhor such a food style and hence, the leaders of a state, if they are using an alkaline, they become popular while exhibiting an alkaline lifestyle.

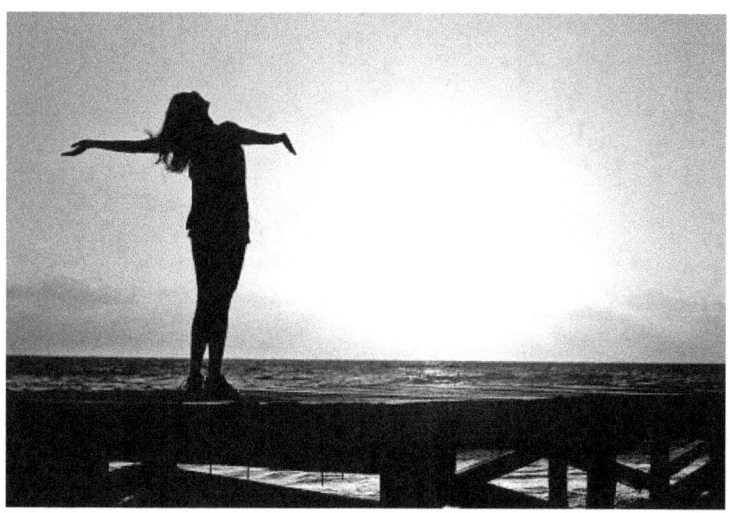

Thus, the modes of working, daily routines and lifestyle are all affected by the proper intake of a fast mimicking diet. Hence, on a social, individualistic and state level, the use of a fast mimicking diet can trigger many bodily changes in a human body, and this is all the cause of the popularity of a fast mimicking diet.

Chapter 9 Which eating protocol to follow

One of the most well-known methods which have been known to facilitate autophagy is intermittent fasting. In this chapter, we will give you seven means of following intermittent fasting. That way, you have a better idea of which method to follow and which you shouldn't.

Seven ways to intermittent fast

Since intermittent fasting has come out, there have been several methods which are being popularized by many fitness experts and gurus. At first, it was the simple fasting strategy which was fast for 16 hours and eat for 8 hours. But since then, we have discovered multiple different ways of fasting which are being used for fat loss and overall well-being.

One of the best things in regard to following intermittent fasting is the ability to have choices. When fasting you have so many ways to go about it that it makes it very user-friendly, as you will learn later on in this chapter. Truthfully if you are deciding to follow intermittent fasting, then you should have no excuse. Intermittent fasting works with you instead of against you unlike most diets out there.

There are many ways to go about fasting, and we will be talking about those in this chapter. Just remember, even though you might have found the right fasting cycle for your lifestyle needs that doesn't mean it will fit your goal. For instance, if your goal is to notice more health benefits from fast rather than weight loss, then there are some fast that works better when compared to other options. Be aware, even though all fasts will help you lose weight and live a healthier life, you still need to make sure that you are following the plan which is right for your needs.

The 12 hours fast

Fasting for 12 hours is one of the ways to get started with fasting. That is the easiest way to learn how fasting works and to figure out how your body reacts to it. Which makes a 12-hour fast an excellent tool for women to find out how their body reacts, and to slowly start to control their hunger cravings?

The 12-hour fast is very simple to follow, and you will be fasting for half the day and eating for half the day. When I put it like that, it doesn't sound so bad, does it?

Although a 12-hour fast is still considered a fast and you will see some benefits from it, it won't be as drastic as something like a 16 hour fast or anything along that line. The 12-hour fast works are great to get your body to prepare for longer fasting and to show you what fasting feels like, it is merely a beginner's tool.

Nonetheless, we highly recommend 12-hour fast for women who are just starting off intermittent fasting. The best way to go about 12 hours fast would be to eat from 8 a.m. till 8 p.m. and then from 8 p.m. to 8 am not eat anything at all, even though this might sound easy for some it will still catch up on you. We recommend you follow the 12-hour fast for four weeks or until you feel like you can fast for a more extended period of time. But, most of the time four weeks does the trick for beginners. Even though, studies are showing that 12-hour fast tends to be the perfect time for fasting as tested on rats.

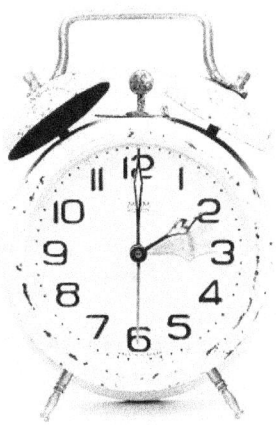

It is still recommended that you fast for a little bit of more extended time, as from personal experience and speaking with other experts in the field of intermittent fasting they recommend ideal fast should be 16 to 20 hours. Regardless when you fast for 12 hours, you'll start to see benefits such as your insulin sensitivity going up your fat loss will kick up a notch, and you will notice more mental focus.

The 12 hours fast does everything right, which makes the 12 hours fast a jack of all trades but a master of none. It is recommended that you only follow this method for a short period to see some results and to get used to fasting; you can pick any time frame you want to fast during. The timings won't make a drastic difference in the type of results you will be getting from the 12 hours fast. As long as you pick a time that works for you, then you should be good.

16 Hour fast

This is the fasting method, which has been popularized to be intermittent fasting. Many people use this method to lose weight and to gain some muscle especially men. But the 16 hours fast has been used successfully by women as well; Martin Berkhan who popularized this method truly lives by it. He has noticed the better fat loss, better health, and more muscle mass by following this plan. Now if putting on muscle is not your goal; the 16 hours fast still has some things to consider.

In one of the newer studies done on obese individuals, they noticed not only fat loss but also reduction and blood pressure. Which means the 16/8 method is excellent for fat loss and lowering the risk of cardiovascular diseases and heart diseases, even though this study was taken part in obese people it is still great to have been backed up by science? Bumping up from 12 hours to 16 hours, you will not notice a big difference in insulin sensitivity and mental focus. But you will see more benefits towards that cellular rejuvenation and better results in fat loss.

You will also notice more detox benefits from the 16 hours fast if compared to the 12 hours, which makes the 16-hour fast a lot more similar to the 12 hours fast. Think of the 16 hours fast as the full version of intermittent fasting whereas the 12-hour fast is the trial version, even though there is only a 4-hour difference between the two it stills makes up for a drastic change.

Once you start fasting for 16 hours instead of 12, you will notice the better fat loss and more health benefits from it. Just like the 12 hours fast, you can follow whichever way you want to pursue this fasting; the timings can be based on your lifestyle. We recommend fasting from 10 pm to 2 pm and eat from 2 pm to 10 pm, but make sure to pick a time that works for you.

Fast for 2 days per week

This fasting method was popularized by Michael Mosley, who is a doctor and journalist. Since this method has no studies to prove its benefits, it is still a method used by many people. Even though this method does not have any solid study to back it up, benefits that are stated include better brain function, Reducing the risk of heart disease, stroke, cancer and improving cholesterol levels.

This method can get tough to follow for some people. However, it will put you in a twenty percent calorie deficit which is a great place to be in if your goal is to lose body fat. This could be an excellent way to lose excess body fat if you can handle it, on that note let's talk about this method and how it works.

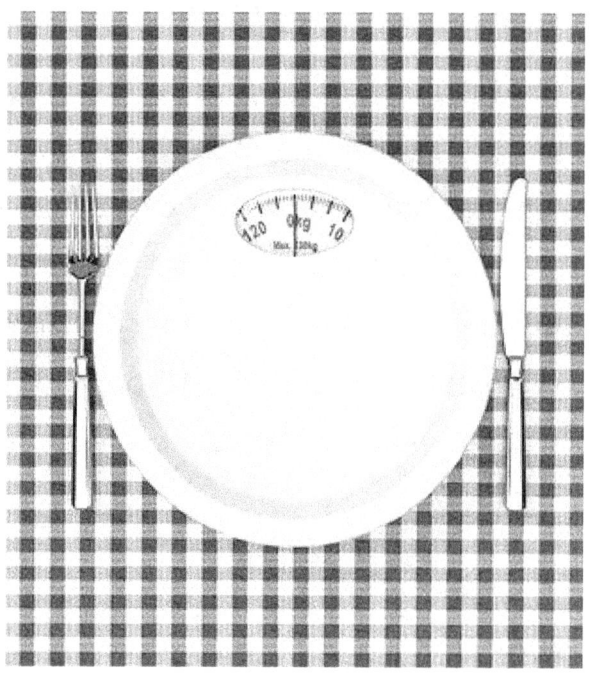

Also known as the 5:2 method is where the person eats an average amount of calories throughout the week and restricts their calories to five hundred/six hundred calories a day for two days. The guideline suggests five hundred calories a day for women and six hundred calories for men on fasting days. The method recommends you have two meals divided into your calories for the day when fasting, which means two meals of two fifty calories for women and two meals of three hundred calories a day for men.

Your calories will not be completely cut out throughout those two days, so make sure you are drinking a ton of water and other no-calorie liquids in between your meals on fasting days. Now the best way that you can go about using this method of fasting would generally be eating through Monday to Friday then fasting over the weekend, and my recommendation would be fast when you don't have work or if you are doing anything physically demanding like working out.

This will ensure you don't feel tired or worst go hypoglycemic as you will be "fasting" for quite a long time, so make sure you are fasting on days you are not working or doing anything physically demanding. Also, the great thing about this method is that there is no food restriction during non-fasting days, which is definitely a good thing for some you foodies out there. Now there are some benefits to these methods, and let's talk about that.

The primary benefit is that you will lose body fat and that too quite quickly, as a result of eating so little during those two days of fasting. I have personally followed this plan just as an experiment and I have to say, and I did lose body fat in those two weeks which I followed it. If your goal is fat loss without restricting your diet as much, then this method can be the one for you.

Another benefit claimed is lower cholesterol, lower risk of heart disease and cancer, which is fantastic for everyone following this method of fasting. But then again, these benefits are claimed, not proven so don't follow this method if your goal is to lower the risk of diseases there are other fasting methods in this book that you can follow to get those benefits. The great thing about this fasting method is that you will get to eat what you want to eat, no need to restrict yourself on non-fasting days but if I were you, I would still be careful. Not to overeat if your goal is to lose body fat, so those are the benefits now let's talk about the cons.

This method is not ideal by any means, there are some flaws to this method, and one of them was used in a positive but it is being used in con. In this method, you can eat whatever you want to eat, which is a flaw since people will eat a lot of junk food as an excuse and not do any justice to their health. I believe that fasting should be accompanied by a well-balanced healthy diet and having junk food on occasion, so I personally don't like the fact of having whatever you want on your non-fasting days as it can take away from the benefits of fasting.

Another flaw of this method is that it can be tough for some people to make it a lifestyle as fasting for two days straight can be a problem, but if it works for you then go for it. The main flaw is that there so no backing up the claims that this method is claiming. Although this is a fasting method and fasting has a lot of benefits that have been backed up, this method doesn't so as I said before don't follow this diet if your sole purpose is to lower the risk of diseases. If you follow a workout plan that requires strength training, then this fasting method might not be the one for you, as this method can hinder your workout quality as it did for some people.

So now you know all about the 5:2 method, this method can be used with great success if your goal is to lose body fat and have basically no restrictions on your diet on non -fasting days. But please use this method for the right reasons; don't use it if you want a lowered risk of diseases as studies have not proved it.

Other fasting methods can be followed if your goal is lower the risks, and if your goal is to get stronger and put on some muscle then this method won't be ideal as this method can affect your workouts. All in all, if this method is being used for the right reasons, then it can lead you to great success in weight loss goals. If this method matches your lifestyle and goals, then follow this fasting protocol. But our recommendation would be to use this plan with a grain of salt and to only use it for a short period. As we don't think this method is a sustainable fasting protocol like the 16/8.

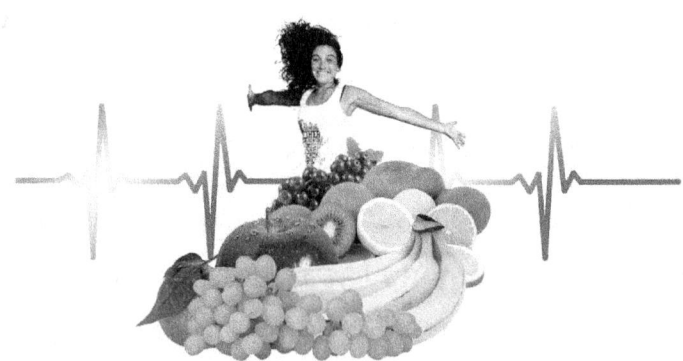

Chapter 10 Professional Guidance During Water-Fasting

With proper medical supervision and adequate guidance, water fasting is an efficient and harmless way of assisting the body in self-restoration. However, like any other thing that affects the body, there are some associated risks. For anyone that is considering undergoing a therapeutic fast, my advice would be to do this under the guidance of a certified IAHP expert who is trained in the process. The International Association of Hygienic Physicians consists of primary care doctors that are experts at supervising therapeutic fasts. Every approved member is a licensed osteopath, medical doctor or chiropractor, that was finalized at least a 6-month residency program at an authorized institution that is specialized in therapeutic fasts. Unlike in the past, fasting is now easily accessible due to the increase in the number of licensed professionals

Advantages of fasting under professional guidance. Maximum health is sustained when the body has adequate health requirements such as proper environment, psychology, and diet. If any of these requirements are inadequate, it affects your health. Most times, therapeutic fasting is an incredibly effective way of health recovery since it enables the body to produce an exceptional response to healing.

No other form of fasting can mimic the benefits of this way of fasting. Fasting, in a busy, noisy, or unsupportive surroundings will deprive the body of the chance to optimize the processes of self-restoration. Total rest is pertinent to optimize the beneficial effects of therapeutic fasting. Drinking juices exclusively or eating particular foods are essential as well. There are tremendous benefits both health and physiologically wise when you consume these foods. However, this does not imply that the elimination diet, otherwise known as the juice diet, is better than straight water fast.

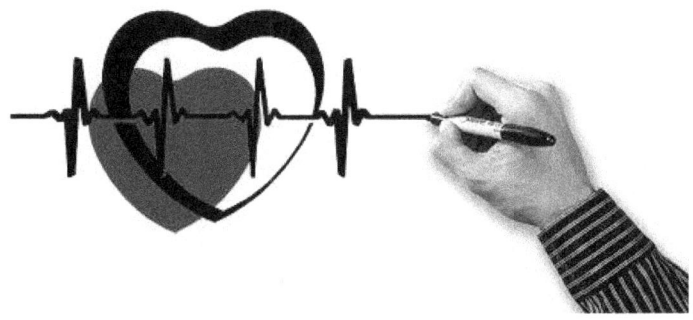

How A Chiropractor Will Help With The Fasting Process

Certain specialists in the health care sector concentrate on recognizing and treating diseases that affect the junction between muscles and nerves, and they are very particular about curing these diseases by molding and sometimes, even altering the spinal cord. These specialists are called Chiropractors.

Chiropractors educate their patients on how to care for themselves by ergonomics, exercising, making user-friendly systems and other remedies to relieve back pain. Their main aim is to lessen the pain felt by patients and to increase their performance.

They believe that periodic fasting purges the body of harmful substances and causes the body to perform optimally.

There are certain criteria chiropractors take heed of during a fast;

First on the list of criteria is preventing death. Chiropractors expect side effects of fasting such as irritability, skin rashes, foul taste in the mouth, headaches, nausea and vomiting, unusual discharges from mucous membranes, postural hypertension and low back pain in the initial stage of fasting as a result of referral activity from kidney changes.

These professionals know that their patients undergo characteristic restorative crisis whereby persistent illnesses develop into short term illnesses and that it can be very distressing. Thus, their responsibility is to detect the boy's attempt to recover through a short-term illness.

They are very mindful of carrying out the proper clinical supervision of their patients, after which they monitor the reaction of the body to the fast to determine the extent and severity of the therapy. To a great length, chiropractors monitor patient's activities like the food they eat, the time they sleep, and even as far as how susceptible they are to levels of stress.

Chiropractors can guarantee a risk-free experience, influencing the slightest reaction to water fasting (including hydration), as a result of the control they have over the patient's activities.

Chapter 11 Which eating pattern will work for you

Now that you're aware of most of the intermittent fasting, we will now help you finalize on what plan you're going to be following when fasting. This chapter will help you realize what works for you when it comes to intermittent fasting because someone 16/8 method might be better suited for some when compared to the 5:2 method. After this chapter, you should be fully equipped to start fasting. Later on, in this book, we will talk about more intermittent fasting related stuff but for now, let us find out which plan to get started with when it comes to intermittent fasting.

<u>Pick a plan</u>

As you could tell, they were all different but none the less effective in their manner. Every fasting method tends to yield different types of results, so it is essential that you picked the right one which works with your lifestyle and your goals. What we will do is go through all the fasting methods step by step and explain to you which one is suited for what type of goals and lifestyle, and after reading those you can decide on which one to start following. If that sounds good let's get started, we will start by talking about the 12 hours fast.

16 hours fast: Very similar to the 12-hour fast, the 16 hour fast is one of the most popular fasting methods used by many. This method is for people who are trying to lose weight, build muscle and live an overall healthy life. If your goal is to get results from autophagy, then this fasting method might be for you, as this is one of the fasting protocols which have been proven to promote autophagy. This plan is ideal for people who are following the 12-hour fast and are looking for a bump, similar effects of the 12-hour fast it is just prolonged for 4 hours. If you're someone looking to get most of the health benefits from intermittent fasting, then this plan is for you. Moreover, if you are someone who demands flexibility with the eating windows, then this plan would be better suited for you.

Fast for 2 days per week: Also known as the 5:2 method, this is one of the more intense fasting protocols. Even though there have been no studies showing the health benefits by following a 5:2 method, it is best known for drastic weight loss. If you're looking to lose weight quickly and efficiently oh, and this plan might be the answer for you. One thing to remember this plan who's better suited for women who had some experience with intermittent fasting, don't start following this plan if you're a complete beginner. This plan can be very easy to cope with on day to day basis, as you can merely fast when you are not working. Overall this plan is excellent for intermediate fasters who are looking to lose weight quickly, and one suggestion would be to not follow this plan for longer than four weeks.

This information should help you tremendously with picking out the fasting protocol for your needs, make sure it is sustainable for you.

Take a look at your diet

Intermittent fasting works excellent, but it works a lot better when you eat healthier overall. For you to achieve better results from intermittent fasting, it needs to be health-focused meals. You see when you start following intermittent fasting alongside a healthy diet, and magic starts to happen. What we will do is give you some pointers on how to begin observing intermittent fasting the right way.

If your goal is to lose body fat your macros should be 40% protein 20% carbs and 40% fats, whereas if your goal is to maintain your weight and reap the benefits of intermittent fasting, then we recommend following a macro protocol of 30% protein 40% carbs and 30% fats. If you want to lose weight, then you need to look at your diet making sure you don't go over your calories and macros. If you aren't eating healthy meals throughout the day, then you can slowly start to incorporate better meals.

Start by having one healthy meal when you break your fast and one meal of whatever you desire, and once you become more comfortable, you can make it two meals. Making you slowly start eating healthier, which will yield even better results overall. Yes, many people do get away with eating foods that aren't healthy, and yes, they so see amazing changes. However, if you want to see over the top changes, then we recommend eating a bit more robust. Now there is no specific diet you need to follow, merely make healthier choices as this should help. You need to take a look at your food which you are eating and make changes where necessary. It will be hard in the beginning but, it will eventually become more natural.

<u>Learn to listen to your body</u>

It's imperative that you listen to your body when you're fasting, listening to your body will help you understand one-stop and will not stop. Intermittent fasting for women can require extra attention, and that is why it is necessary to listen to your body. There are some telltale signs to look out for when doing intermittent fasting, know that most of the symptoms should subside within a week.

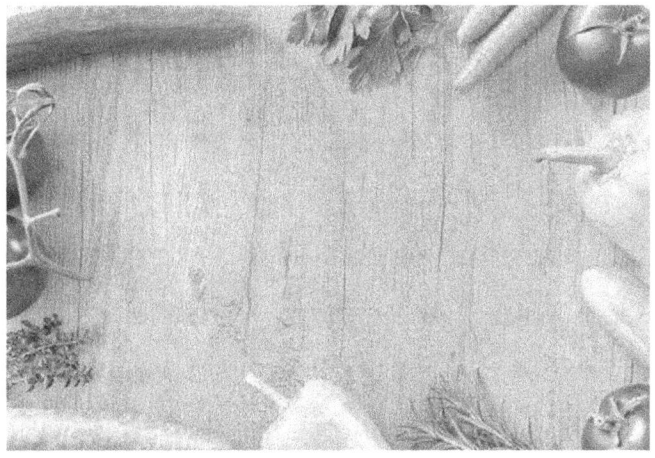

However, if they don't chance are you need to switch up your fasting protocol. One of the ways to tell the intermittent fasting is becoming way too hard for you, is when you start feeling cold chronically. Once you begin to feel cold chronically, that's a big sign that intermittent fasting is becoming very hard for you to follow if you feel cold throughout the day for three weeks plus then chances are it is time for you to lower the fasting

intensity. Another sign to consider when you're intermittent fasting would be the extreme hunger.

In the first couple of weeks you will feel extreme hunger, but if that keeps happening for over three weeks chances are your body is telling you that you can't follow intermittent fasting at this level. These are the significant signs you need to listen to your body when intermittent fasting, but always make sure you get your blood work done and get the professional help if you feel like intermittent fasting is affecting you physically. Best rules to live by when intermittent fasting if it doesn't feel right three weeks into it then stop. Nonetheless, symptoms could occur anytime, just be in-tuned with your body and make sure you are listening to it.

Helpful tips dealing with hunger

When following an intermittent fasting routine, it is crucial that you make sure that your appetite is under control to make sure fast isn't broken prematurely. Time and time again, many followers of the intermittent fasting have broken the fast prematurely just because they couldn't control their hunger. We will go multiple ways to deal with hunger, and overall help you continue with intermittent fasting. The first tip is pretty obvious, and that is to drink more water. Much of the time, hunger is thirst.

Meaning you will be able to control your eating desires by drinking more water, having more water through the day helps you tremendously to control your hunger. Another method for managing your hunger would be to drink more coffee and green tea, and caffeine has shown to suppress hunger which overall helps you with fasting. Just make sure the coffee or tea you drink does not contain any sugar or milk, as that could break your fast. Getting yourself busy will help you control your hunger, most of the time when we occupy our self with work, we tend to forget the food.

Perhaps do some work, or household chores to keep yourself busy when you feel like eating. You can also exercise or go for a walk, and this will kill two birds with one stone. When you start walking, you will take your mind of fasting, and you will also burn some fat while doing so. If you are feeling more energetic, then you can go ahead and get a full workout. However, remember that you might feel hungry after the workout if you have no experience in managing your hunger. Now, if you are looking for a more relaxed way of managing your hunger, then we would recommend meditation.

Meditation works well when it comes to controlling your hunger, and it will also help you manage your mental stress if you have any. Make sure you are using this tool, to manage your hunger, and who knows you might really enjoy meditation. The final technique we recommend would be to eat more fibrous foods before you start your fast, as this will help you stay fuller for a long period of time. Many followers of intermittent fasting will eat junk food, this will actually make them crave foods faster than someone who ate a good healthy meal with a ton of fiber in it.

If you want to have a better less hungry fasting window, then we highly recommend you eat healthy meals with a ton of fiber in them before you start fasting. These are all the tips and tricks to dealing with hunger, make sure that you are following all these tips to control your hunger when fasting. Especially if it is your first three weeks fasting, as that is when you will notice most of the hunger cravings. These tips will help you tremendously to power through those first three weeks and help you with completing your fast.

Track your progress

If you want to be successful with intermittent fasting, then you need to start tracking your progress. Tracking your progress is the main reason why most people continue on with intermittent fasting and why most people don't, and there's a reason for that. You see, when you start tracking your daily progress, you will begin to notice better results which will help you hold yourself accountable to it. There are three ways to track your progress when intermittent fasting, and we will talk about those today. The first way you can track your progress is

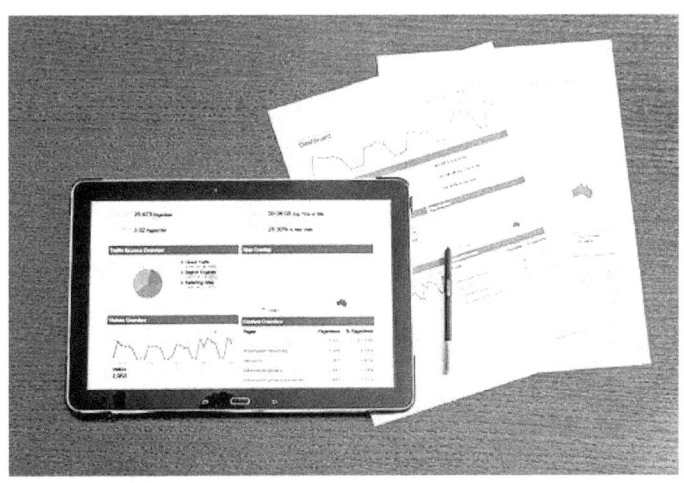

by daily journaling, write down everything how you felt and how your body was feeling when fasting.

Not only will this teach you how to listen to your body, but it would also show your progress so if you're ever feeling down you can just go back and read past experiences and results with intermittent fasting and see how much better you have gotten. Another method to track your fasting would be to schedule out your whole week in terms of time frame like when it comes to fasting and eating window. Most people just go day-by-day fasting whenever they feel, which is fine, but you'll see much better results if you figure out your whole week, so set up your fasting windows and eating windows.

This method would also help you stay accountable for your fasting goals. The third way to track your progress would be to measure your body composition every week. This will not only keep you motivated in terms of keeping you moving forward, but it would also help you see how you're progressing, and if changes are needed to be made. These are the three main ways to track your progress and to stay on track with intermittent fasting, and we recommend using all three.

Remember that most people give up or quit because they don't have a plan or a strategy to get somewhere. Once you start tracking your progress and tracking your intermittent fasting schedules, you will notice that you are a lot more accountable with your goals and you will begin to see better results.

We highly recommend you start tracking your progress and especially use these tools that we just talked about. There are also apps, which can be used to track your progress. If you don't like writing stuff out, then you can download apps that will help you to track your progress. Overall there should be no excuse not to track your progress. Also, we recommend you journal your body composition weekly and your journaling daily.

The journaling works a lot better when written daily since your emotions are at its peak when you write them out. However, if you feel that daily journaling can become hard, you can also journal weekly. Nonetheless, daily journaling is a lot better. Follow whatever feels best for you but remember to track all three progress to see better results, it doesn't matter how you track it as long you track it.

Chapter 12 The Importance of Detox

Our bodies can detox themselves through natural processes in the livers, kidneys, skin, and bowels and through autophagy. However, we can also take special steps to detox ourselves through our diets and other lifestyle changes. This chapter is dedicated to the reasons why you might want to consider taking further steps to detox yourself.

Detox diets have earned a reputation of being based upon frivolous pseudoscience, but detoxing is an incredibly important process in our body. Our health is assaulted from all angles by toxins and pollutants; everything from caffeine and alcohol to air pollutants from industrial waste, car exhaust, and cigarette smoke. Most of the things we eat, even foods we consider healthy, have small amounts of toxic substances within them. Yet we can also allow toxins to enter our bloodstream through the skin and through the air that enters our lungs. Regardless of their source, our body regularly needs to deal with all the nasty compounds and chemicals that end up in the body, otherwise, we can face corresponding nasty health consequences.

In the body, the liver and the kidneys are the organs responsible for dealing with toxins in the body. The kidneys filter toxins from the blood, whilst the liver breaks down toxins into substances that can be used by the body or passed without trouble. If the kidneys and liver are burdened with too many toxins or if they are not kept in good shape through a healthy lifestyle, they can be unable to deal with all the toxins in the body. This can cause a huge array of problems; anything from fatigue and general feelings of being unwell to bloating and digestive problems and even liver disease.

Most detox diets are aimed at eating lots of foods that help keep the liver and kidney in tip-top shape, but there are also many other methods to keep these crucial organs healthy. Drinking lots of water – at least 6 to 8 glasses per day – allows any waste products of the liver and kidneys to easily pass through the body. Likewise, you should avoid smoking and second-hand cigarette smoke, which contains over 4,000 different chemicals, including 43 cancer-causing carcinogens.

Eating too much sugar also makes your liver unhappy. By now everyone knows how consuming too much sugar can contribute to diabetes and the various health issues associated with weight gain, but the effects of sugar on the liver remain an enigma to most. The liver has a very limited ability to metabolize sugar, with some dieticians suggesting that anything more than 6 teaspoons of added sugar is excessive. Any sugar that the liver cannot break down is stored as fat, and a build-up of fat in the liver can lead to a condition called fatty liver disease.

Fatty liver disease, in turn, can lead to more serious conditions as bodily pain, fatigue, weakness and cirrhosis of the liver. Most people who are overweight or obese are at increased risk of fatty liver disease and they may be suffering from the condition in its early stages when there are few explicit symptoms.

Caffeine is another common toxin that the body has to deal with regularly. Caffeine is commonly associated with coffee, but it is also present in most fizzy drink's chocolate and energy drinks. The liver interprets caffeine as a foreign chemical and it is broken down through a special pathway in the liver that deals with manmade and unfamiliar substances, which includes most medication. For this reason, heavy caffeine consumption should especially be avoided when also taking certain drugs, especially pain relief chemicals such as acetaminophen.

Moderate caffeine consumption isn't dangerous or even unhealthy, with some studies suggesting it has numerous benefits on the body. Nonetheless, for the purposes of cleansing the body of toxins and giving the liver a period of relief, it's best to avoid this energy-booster or at least cut down on your silent addiction.

Good liver health can also be maintained by eating a diet rich in antioxidants which aid in processing the waste products of toxins. Common antioxidants include vitamin C, vitamin E, beta-carotene, and zinc. Foods that are rich in antioxidants include dark chocolate, legumes, blueberries, red grapes, nuts, dark green veg, orange vegetable, and green tea.

You can also help detox through eating organic food whenever possible. Non-organic foods are free from pesticide residue that may be left on non-organic foods. Many pesticides can build up in the human body and may be dangerous in noticeable concentrations. Eating organic, however, isn't always possible, practical or affordable, so sometimes it may be necessary to compromise. In general, if you eat the outer surface of grown food, it's more important that it is organic. Fruit such as strawberries, apples, grapes, cherries, and leafy greens should preferably be organic, whereas with fruit or veg with peel it is less important (such as bananas and onions). The easiest way to detox your body is always to avoid toxins in the first place!

There is also a detox method you might not expect; getting more sleep. The western world has an embarrassing relationship with sleep. Sleep is vital for our well-being in dozens of different ways – it's where we rest our minds and rejuvenate our body. Yet all too many people resent their need to sleep and try to cheat themselves out of an hour or two every night. This can take a serious toll on well-being.

In terms of detoxing and cleansing the body, most of the detox process occurs during sleep. In the resting state of sleep, your body is free to use resources and act in ways it simply can't when you are awake. For example, one of the main purposes of sleep is to filter toxins out of the brain; toxins which naturally as a side effect of being awake. The filtering system is called the lymphatic system and it is thought to be 10 times more activated during sleep, than during wakefulness. During sleep, numerous other metabolic processes take part, such as those which occur in the liver and are inhibited whilst active.

Whilst it might be rather obvious it is also worth mentioning that you can prevent toxins from getting into your system by avoiding places and environments where there are toxins present. Exhaust fumes, second-hand smoke and low air quality from industrial pollution are the main culprits but depending on your location and career you may come into contact with many other types of toxins such as chemical residue from working in a factory, for example.

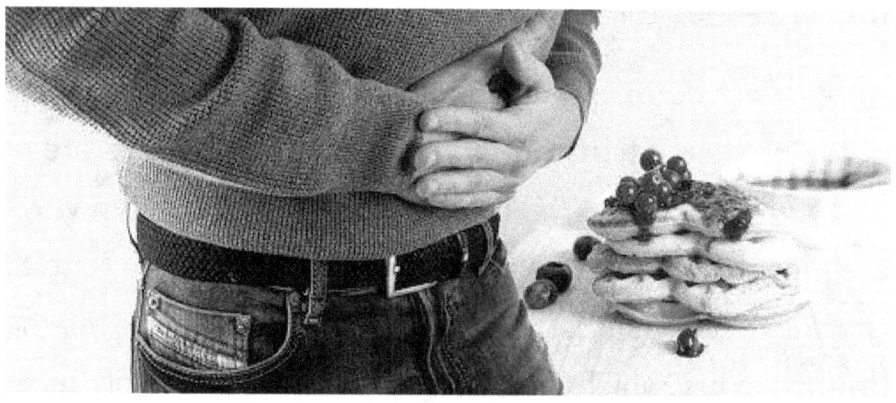

You can also aid the detox process by taking certain supplements, most notably milk thistle. Milk thistle is a small plant that grows in Mediterranean regions. It can be used as a herb and it also goes by the names Mary

Thistle or Holy Thistle. Milk thistle is a popular natural choice for helping treat liver conditions such as cirrhosis or jaundice and it is also a staple of the detox community.

The active ingredient in milk thistle is called silymarin and it has powerful anti-inflammatory properties as well as being an antioxidant. Research on silymarin is still progressing and it's not entirely clear how it affects the body. Some studies have suggested that silymarin can aid liver function in individuals who have been exposed to industrial toxins, such as xylene and there is evidence to help it also improves type 2 diabetes and lowers cholesterol.

Finally, you can also try a temporary cleansing diet. Ultimately, our body needs the right materials to detox and as you might now understand, our regular diets don't give us enough resources to work with. You can rectify this by trying a cleansing diet intended to give your body a huge boost of all the vitamins, minerals, and good stuff it needs to cleanse itself.

Of course, ideally, a healthy, balanced diet will help the body cleanse itself over time and be exposed to fewer toxins. However, whether it's due to personal fault or factors beyond our control, we can't always consume a perfectly healthy diet. It might just be too pricey; we might not have the time, or we might constantly be around other people who influence or control our eating habits.

Therefore, as a temporary solution or as a compromise you can periodically embrace a cleansing detox diet. These types of diets aren't intended to be a permanent change to your eating patterns, and you shouldn't follow them for any period longer than 1-week. However, with that being said, they can give your body a reprieve to repair and rejuvenate itself, a benefit that can last for a few weeks or months before being required once more.

There are many different types of cleansing and detox diets, most of which involve consuming a large amount of fruit, vegetables, and calorie-free drinks. Try one out for a week and see how you feel afterward!

Eat Probiotics!

If you decide to detox it might seem like the list of prohibited foods is huge. However, there are still many great choices for a detox diet, and you should still find that you can eat a diverse and tasty diet during your detox and body cleanse.

In particular, *probiotics* are a good choice. Probiotics are a group of foods that contain 'good' bacteria that promote a healthy gastrointestinal ecosystem. As you may know, your gut contains tens of thousands of different bacteria, some of which can benefit your health, some which cause harm and some which have little impact. The health of the bowels is increasingly understood to be crucial to human health, with some studies suggesting that the flora of the gut influencing how many nutrients and calories you absorb from your food and even contributing to mood swings and depressions. In fact, probiotics have also been argued to help prevent diarrhea, gut disease, and improve eczema although the support for these claims is controversial.

There are many different probiotic foods, including yogurt, sauerkraut, miso soup, kefir, sourdough bread, and tempeh, all of which are considered healthy detox-friendly foods, at least when eaten in moderation. Probiotics can also be found as a supplement, although if you decide to take a specific probiotic supplement it's worth further researching what the proposed benefits are – there are many different types of probiotic supplement all of the different supposed effects.

Changing your Eating Habits

Whether you are attempting a detox diet or trying to fast, you are not only working against your natural instinct to eat but any habits and emotions that revolve around food. You might eat when you are tired to give you a boost in energy, binge to perk up your mood or make poor choices just out of routine or mindlessness. Regardless of your reasons for a detox diet or a fast to work, you need to control how you interact with food.

Start by thinking about your current habits. Are you an emotional eater? Do you like to reward yourself with food? The first stage to overcoming these habits is simply recognizing them and being honest with yourself. It's better to admit your faults rather than to pretend that they don't exist; they'll be there regardless.

By acknowledging how you interact with the food you can anticipate and prepare for any temptations that occur during your fast or detox. By depriving yourself of food or by forcing yourself to eat a cleansing diet, you will encounter these feelings and they will probably be stronger than they usually are.

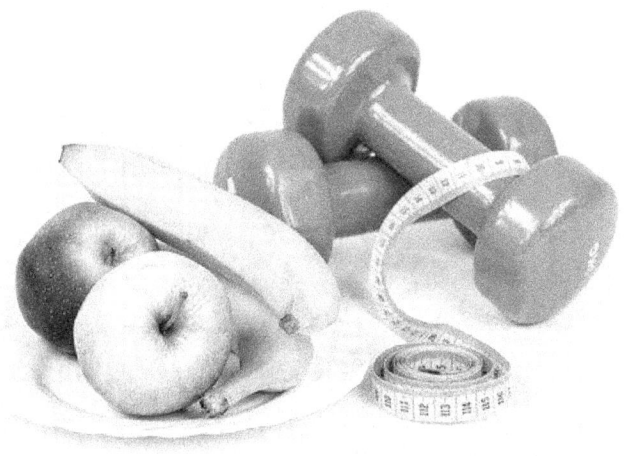

Learn to challenge your feelings and your thoughts. Are you really hungry? Do you really need to give up on your fast? Isn't there an alternative, more productive way to deal with your emotions? Try meditating or doing some activities, such as walking your dog or tackling a task you've been putting off. By engaging with an activity, you consider positive you'll feel much better afterward and the emotions that were bothering you will dissipate.

Also, learn to just sit and be comfortable with your feelings. Instead of shying away from the emotional pain that might be driving you to binge eat, or simply the lack of motivation to continue, take a moment to pause in your day and explore these feelings. Are they strong or weak? How do they affect your thought patterns? How are these feelings affecting your body – can you explore where these feelings are actually occurring? The more you learn to delve into these feelings instead of running away, the more mundane they will become and the less influence they will have over you.

You should also make an effort to be mindful of your eating patterns, in both a detox diet and an eating pattern that involves fasting. You might find that you gorge on your food without truly considering or tasting it, or when you come home from work you automatically start browsing around in the fridge for something to snack on. By trying to be more aware of your interactions with food, you can help manage temptations and habits that urge you to eat.

Finally, try to think positively about your detox diet or fast. Studies have shown that it's easier to change your habits by developing positive habits, rather than breaking negative habits. Or in other words, instead of thinking 'I want to stop feeling so lethargic and bloating it's better to think 'I want to be successful in my detox diet'. These two thoughts might relate to the same goal, but the latter has a much more positive vibe to it, which also makes it easier to strive towards.

Dealing with Other People

Many people won't appreciate the benefits of fasting or a detox diet. You can cite a hundred different studies or try to explain your motivations as logically and clearly as possible, but people might still sneer or disregard what you are doing.

As a result, it's best to consider carefully who you talk about your diet. Do they need to know? Does it bother you if you don't have their approval? It might not be a big deal if someone doesn't accept your diet, but it can still make your life easier if you are not listening to snide comments or objections every time you are around them.

You can always find support online or a detox and fasting community nearby to talk to. These people will understand and be more welcoming. Of course, you may be fortunate to be surrounded by friends and family who are considerate, or at the very least, appreciate what you are doing is important to you.

If you have to tell people, just try and be as clear and reasonable about the discussion as possible. Laying a strong foundation for why you are doing a fast or detox diet will help people accept it; if your first explanation is watertight, people will find it hard to object, yet if you explain yourself poorly, you'll be dogged by criticism throughout.

Chapter 13 Regulation of inflammation and improved muscle performance by autophagy

It is the preservation of life when the body is working to fight off something in times of stress or even starvation. These microscopic performance activates to repair the cells and any damage that could be caused by illness and inflammation. This process can also deplete or starve unwanted intruders from the vital nutrients they need to survive, allowing for their death and renewal.

The benefits of autophagy are limitless and can change your body function deep down on the cellular level. Some benefits are:

- Promotion of a longer, healthier life through cell regeneration
- *Helps in weight loss by encouraging healthier metabolism*—Autophagy can help clean and restore the toxic accumulation in the mitochondria, the energy makers of the cell. This is where fat gets burned and Adenosine Triphosphate (ATP) is produced. ATP is the compound that provides certain cellular energy,

specifically muscle contraction. Autophagy allows for greater efficiency to boost metabolism and energy stores.

- *Risks of neurodegenerative disease are decreased* Diseases in the brain take a long time to occur and happen over time with the buildup of misfolded, old, or dysfunctional proteins in or around the brain cells. The chemical compounds linked to the cause of Parkinson's disease, synuclein, is removed through autophagy. Studies suggest that the same may be true in cases of Alzheimer's, removing the compound amyloid from the brain that is known to be associated with this disease. Another neurodegenerative disease is dementia caused by diabetes. Chronic insulin resistance disallows autophagy from occurring so no clean up can occur within the cell, leaving them in a toxic wasteland of malfunction.

- *Regulation of inflammation*—Autophagy allows inflammation when it is needed to fight off invaders, yet also reduces inflammation when it is the chronic response to over-triggered signals to the cells and the body.

- Helps fight infectious disease
- *Improves muscle performance*—Muscles undergo stress during exercise. Microscopic tearing in the fibers of muscles occurs during strenuous activity. The muscle fibers, also made of specific kinds of cells, are repaired through the process of autophagy. Over time, as you build muscle, it will reduce the amount of energy needed to utilize the muscle in general.
- *Prevents the onset of cancer*—Though research is still being done to understand the effects of autophagy on various kinds of cancer, studies have indicated that it can help to prevent cancer from forming. Scientists who have studied the impact of impaired autophagy response in mice see an uprise of cancer in the mice. To perform the study, the mice involved had their autophagic response mechanism cut off from fully functioning. The result was cancer. The question is, can it work as a treatment for cancer, instead of just preventing it through autophagy? How would inducing autophagy impact other treatments? More

research must be done to understand the impact of induced autophagy in pre-existing cancer treatments like chemotherapy, but it may be that it could have a greater benefit than chemo which can be incredibly damaging to the body if applied long term.

- *Improvement in digestive health*—Autophagy is activated through fasting for short periods intermittently. The break from calorie intake and digestion alone can help your digestive system immensely; everyone needs a break now and then. More to that, while your body is resting from needing to digest, the cells that make up your digestive system and all other systems in your body will be activated to perform autophagy because of the fast, leading to a purification of the cells.

- *Improves the health of the skin*—damage from sun exposure, toxins in the air, changes in temperature, acute ailments like bruises, scrapes, punctures, and burns may all benefit from the autophagic performance. While you may be constantly replacing cells, autophagy keeps the cells fresh and renewed, giving a glow to the skin.

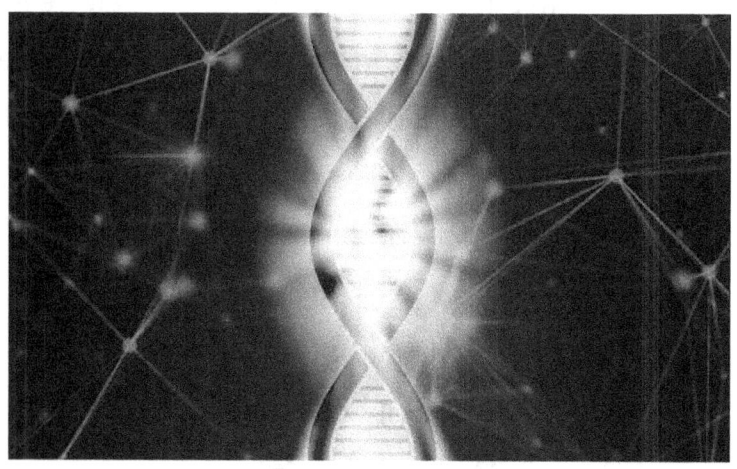

-

- *Minimizes cell death or apoptosis*—With autophagy functioning, the cells are constantly being cleaned and rejuvenated; without it, the cells are piling up with waste and eventually struggle to perform well, leading to a programmed death of the cell. When that

- happens, the cell leaves behind trash that needs to be taken out, and if the cell itself is dead, autophagy won't occur because the process occurs inside the cell. The body will have to trigger an inflammatory response to clean up the cell death aftermath.

- *Improved cognition, memory, and brain function*—Autophagy enhances neuroplasticity, the brain's ability to form and reorganize synaptic connections. There is an increase in cognitive ability through the increase of mitochondria. When your brain cells can function well, so can your whole brain.

- Regulation of hormones, which allows for overall body high performance and function.

- *Improves cardiovascular health*—Autophagy works to clean toxins and biowaste from the cells of the heart muscle, which is constantly pumping blood through your whole body. Aiding in the general renewal of these cells brings about a better functioning heart.

The list goes on, and discoveries about the effects of autophagy on the health of the body continue to demonstrate the beneficial impact of the autophagic performance. When you create opportunities to enhance and promote autophagy, you are enhancing and promoting the health of every cell in your body.

Risks and Cautions of Performance Autophagy

Before you move ahead and begin the process of activating autophagy, it is important to be aware of cautions and risks. To have the best benefit from creating this healing response, you need to plan ahead and be informed about how to do it properly so that you don't cause yourself harm.

There are three main ways that you will learn to activate autophagy in this book: exercise, ketosis, and fasting. When covering the risks, you will understand what can happen or potentially go wrong while using these methods to activate autophagy. Bear in mind that if you are suffering from any severe medical issues, chronic illness, or disease, then it is always a good idea to consult a doctor before beginning this process.

This chapter will briefly cover some of the risks and precautions in initiating autophagy so that you can be prepared to plan your experience well.

Some risks and precautions:

- *Losing the wrong kind of weight*—If you lose muscle instead of fat, you are losing the wrong kind of weight. If you don't need to lose a lot of fat through diet, or fasting, then you have to ensure that you consume enough fat prior to fasting. Your body must be prepared to enter a period without calorie intake, and if you have no fat to burn, then you may find yourself losing some muscle. This is not usually the case if you are fasting properly, preparing in advance, and giving your body time to rest while you are on the fast. Some people will try to do intense exercise on a fast to create an even greater increase in the autophagic response. This is when your body will start to turn to the protein of your body for energy. Make sure you are approaching fasting to induce autophagy healthily.
- *Dehydration*—during intermittent water fast, you may run the risk of dehydration. Fasting is taking a break from food and food contains a percentage of your daily water intake. You will

- need to make sure you are drinking the right amount of water to stay hydrated. On the other hand, drinking too much water can drown the cells, and drinking too much too fast can lead to hyponatremia which is the loss of sodium in the body. Loss of salt in your body can lead to an extreme drop in blood pressure. Drop-in sodium levels due to excess water will cause fluid shifts from outside to inside the cell. The swell causes pressure in the skull which can lead to headaches, nausea, and vomiting. Severe cases of decreased blood pressure can lead to confusion, problems breathing, sleepiness, confused state, weakened muscles, and cramping.

- *Urge to overeat after fasting*—Returning to food after a fast must be done slowly, in steps. When you are not healthily performing a fast, you may be inclined to overeat following the fasting period. If done regularly, this can have a detrimental impact on the body, causing shock to your system.

- Extreme fasting can lead to starvation and eventually death

- *If you fast for too long your body will start to eat itself*—If you are performing a fast for an extreme length of time without any calories, or supplements, your body will start to eat muscle, including cardiovascular muscle and also cells like brain cells. This can be avoided by choosing the right length of time for you're fast, the right fast for your needs, and the right mineral and vitamin supplement to aid the process and prevent muscle loss. There is an important window of benefit for creating autophagy in a fast—between activation and the point where your body stops burning fat and starts eating muscle.

- *Loss of vitamins and minerals from food can cause health problems*—It is important to allow a mineral supplement. Since there are no calories in many supplements, you will not be breaking the fast, although some vitamins can cause discomfort in the stomach if not taken with food, so finding the right vitamins is important for fasting comfort.

- *Less serious, but important precautions and risks is the effect on mood*—Irritability, moodiness, highs and lows, energy depletion, low blood pressure, and dizziness.

- *Improper fasting can raise stress hormone levels-* If you are not engaging in fasting properly, you may encounter the issue of increased stress hormones in the body which isn't good for long periods and can be very damaging to many systems.

- *Fast detoxifying can impact your health*—The rate of detox when fasting is rapid. Toxins held in your body fat for long periods will release in your bloodstream as your body burns fat for calorie consumption. Too many toxins in the bloodstream can feel terrible and lead to nausea, sickness, and a general unwell feeling.

- *A fasting high can impact your cognitive ability*—Sometimes during a fast, you may experience fasting high, a feeling of euphoria as your body shifts and heals. Sometimes, this mental state can make it challenging for you to reasonably listen to your body, making sure you are not overdoing it.

A majority of the risks and precautions can be easily

avoided if you approach autophagic performance with knowledge and preparation. Because the benefits of autophagy are so powerful, it is worth experiencing. With the right diet, exercise, fasting, and rest, you can healthfully activate autophagy safely and beneficially.

Conclusion

Based on what you have learned so far, it is easy to see why many health experts consider autophagy as the key to extending human lifespan. It is also aligned with the main guiding principles of other diets, fitness regimens, and even religious groups. Autophagy is all about achieving the balance between the different metabolic cycles going on within the body.

It may seem confusing and overwhelming at this point, especially considering the various lifestyle changes that you can apply to improve your health and activate autophagy. To get over this, remember that at the end of the day, you are free to choose how much and what will you change about yourself.

Start little by little but maintain consistency in what you decide to do. By doing this, autophagic practices would gradually become incorporated into your personal habits. Doing them would feel more natural, and you would be able to carry them out without even having to think much about what you are supposed to do next, or why you should be doing it in the first place.

Please note that you should not put this off. If you want to live a healthier and longer life, then you have to start working on attaining your goals as soon as possible. There is no better than when you first understood how you can turn your dreams into reality. What you have learned from this book would still be fresh in your mind, and your motivation to further increase your knowledge about autophagy would be at its peak.

Avoid placing your hope in external factors that claim to be capable of combatting or even reversing the aging process. As proven by the numerous studies about autophagy, your body is perfectly capable of doing this as long as you are willing to commit to religious practicing the autophagic methods you have chosen for yourself. You might be tempted to go for a miracle supplement that would boost your longevity, or you might be inclined to wait for medical advances in the field of biohacking and genetic modifications. It is alright to entertain those thoughts, but, at this point, these methods are largely untested or theoretical at best.

Lastly, do not think that reading this book is sufficient

enough for you to be an expert in autophagy. There is so much you can learn through more research ad readings about autophagy, and through practical experience. You should also respect the nuances and complexities of your body. What works for you today may not work at all, or maybe even be harmful to you, the following day.

I'd like to thank you and congratulate you for transiting my lines from start to finish.

I hope this book was able to help you to understand the main principles and guidelines about autophagy.

The next step is to determine the current status of health, and from there, establish your fitness and longevity goals. This is important because you cannot simply adopt the diet or training program of another person, thinking that the outcome would be the same. Take the time to assess yourself first before making any changes to the way you live.

I wish you the best of luck!

www.ingramcontent.com/pod-product-compliance
Lightning Source LLC
Chambersburg PA
CBHW070338220526
45467CB00001B/167